The Real Drama: Incredible Medicine

Pepi Granat, MD

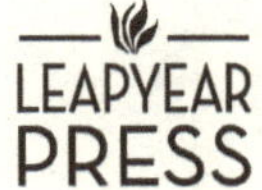

LEAPYEAR
PRESS

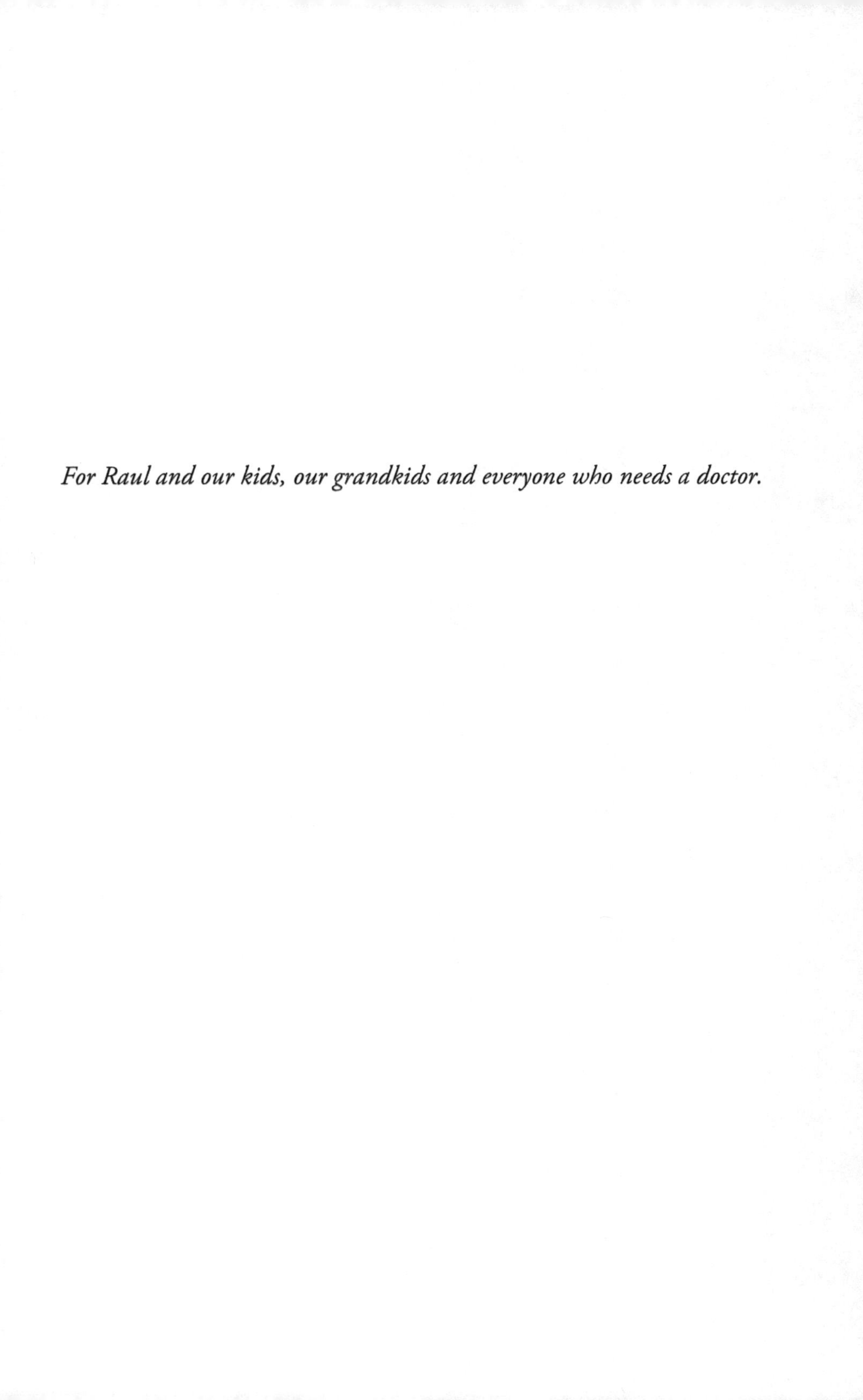

For Raul and our kids, our grandkids and everyone who needs a doctor.

Table of Contents

Foreword

This is a book to pique the interest of doctors and patients because they can glean insights into the lives of patients recounted, and garner points of view they might find of merit. There is a reason that television shows depicting medical doctors in action, both medically and in their private lives, are some of the most watched programs. Medicine is fascinating, riveting, in all its aspects. Doctors will recognize themselves here; patients may relate to their experiences in medicine, whether ill themselves, or aiding a friend or loved one. The quasi-political viewpoints raised here will be of interest to those with strong opinions, either to agree or vehemently dissent. Those with no opinions or who are "on the fence" may want to reexamine and reconsider some of these issues.

This book will show, by personal example, how dilemmas of patient care that affect the larger society can lead to action and change, spearheaded by concerned doctors, with help from interested, involved others. It's my hope to shed some light on why the generalist approach to patient care, with liberal use of specialist expertise when indicated, is best suited to taking good care of patients throughout their lives. Fragmented, poor quality care will result if we allow the generalist to fade into obscurity because of shortsighted disincentives. We will have glimpses into the personal maladies, tragedies and triumphs of patients and doctors, and show how important and how special individual relationships can be, and how they comprise the patchwork quilt and thus the quality and integrity of the whole fabric.

During six decades as a doctor, still in active practice, I have seen many patients whose maladies are traceable to unresolved societal problems.

These issues range from the evils of tobacco to the medical malpractice mess, from drowning prevention to keeping medicine free from religious infringement, especially for women. Certain of these causes called for activism. Many of our medical colleagues have done heroic work in organizations and volunteer efforts, some of which I've been privileged to participate in, some of which I've initiated. Sometimes I have tilted at windmills, virtually alone, often uselessly, but sometimes with dramatic and positive results. Telling these stories may help others realize that they can effect change, too.

If we deplore our medical system when it doesn't serve our needs, we have the power to seek to understand it, and to change it. I want to share some insights gleaned and distilled over those decades in medicine. I hope I have grown and changed, professionally and personally, through each experience.

We would all be happier and healthier with a medical system (or "non-system," as it were) that meets our needs better. While this book is partly about our medical world, it is also about the world of patients and the active practice of medicine and how their care and cure fits into the lives of their doctors.

Why write this book? I wrote this book for the same reason people give for climbing a tall mountain: because it was there.

It was there in two ways: First, the challenge was there of communicating an individual point of view that I know is shared by many of my colleagues, patients, friends and others, and I believe will be shared by many more, once they come to see things in a slightly different light than is usually presented in the confusing media and messages we receive. I refer mainly to the pending disappearance of the true generalist physician and the peril this poses for people everywhere, but also to the abridgement of freedom for doctors and patients, by commerce and government. This change in point of view could lead to a more realistic and beneficial outlook for individual physicians and patients, and for our entire medical system.

Second, a lot of this book has already been written. It was my privilege to have been named editor of *Miami Medicine*, a monthly medical journal, the official organ of the Miami-Dade County Medical Association, from 1992-1995. During those years I selected an editorial board among colleagues who showed interest in writing or in obtaining writers for articles. We worked diligently to put out a well-rounded view of many different themes in medicine, for which we obtained authoritative authors. Most of these themes had little to do with the technical content or subject of medicine, but were universal themes such as aging, non-medical pursuits by doctors, death and dying, innovation and research, doctors' offspring becoming doctors, medical systems around the world, violence as a public health problem, history and medicine, music and medicine, etc.

For each themed issue, I wrote an editorial pertinent to the theme. I was gratified to have received very positive feedback both from colleagues, and lay persons who read these essays. Many people suggested that others would like to read them and that I publish all or most of them. So, in a sense, the book was there all along. I made sure to retain the copyright to these pieces. I have published other articles—both scientific and non-scientific—in a number of other journals and publications who have kindly granted me permission to add them to this collection.

Although one physician's experience could not represent everyone else's, my forty-year sojourn in general medicine has led to some musings, observations and viewpoints that resonate with many of my colleagues and patients. The "public," which includes all of us together, will make decisions for the future of medicine as a profession, and for their own medical care. We will do this by how we vote, how we pay attention to issues, how we value and pay for our care. That is to say, how we think about doctors, patients and medical care will decide what happens to us, as individuals and as a society. We are all responsible for the patchwork quilt that is our medical care, and for its ultimate strength and quality.

This book will pull together disparate, yet integrated musings, activities and stories. There will be, sprinkled among discrete themes, the real meat of medicine—patients. There will be poignant, sad, thrilling, and appalling true stories of patients that either illustrate a point, or are interesting, illuminating or uplifting. There will also be fleeting glimpses into one woman's private world of family, of medicine and of family medicine with some of the events that shaped her daily life and medical world view.

I offer this book with the simple hope that medical students, young and older physicians, patients and others will take heart that you can "fight city hall" and win, that we can all get the medical care and the system we need, and that one can be healthy and happy in a medical career.

Prologue: Against the Tree

The brakes screeched for longer than they should have and then the impact resounded through the neighborhood. I heard steel and glass crunching and breaking, then dead silence except for a spinning sound that could have been the motor. Then I could hear people shrieking, all in the space of less than a minute. It sounded as though it was right outside my door. I had been unpacking boxes in the garage, while my three children, under three-and-a-half, played in their rooms, the baby in the crib for a nap.

As my heart leapt in my chest, I knew I had no choice but to try to help. This had to be serious trauma, just from the sound of it. I was barefoot, wearing a ratty housedress. I didn't even know the neighbors—we had just moved in a month or two before. I dropped the boxes and ran outside to the street's edge, just to see where and what it was. It was right across the street, at the house next door to the one opposite our house. A small, red, two-door Chevette had plunged into a tree at high speed, negotiating the bend that is our street, and was stuck in the tree on a slant, the driver's side smashed into the tree. One of the wheels was still spinning. I was torn between running to see what I could do, and protecting the children. I caught sight of a neighbor I had barely just met, and ran up to her to tell her in a low voice that I was a doctor, and would see to the wreck, but could she watch the kids for a minute? I knew the baby was safe in the crib, but the three and a half old and the two year old were another story. I really didn't want them to see too much of the trauma either. The neighbors had all called 911 and police sirens could be heard in the distance, all in the space of two or three minutes.

There were four young women in the car, two in front, two in back. Later we heard there was wine in brown bags. The driver was slumped against the huge tree trunk, a large banyan, wedged so tightly that she couldn't be reached at all from the driver's side, and barely from the passenger side, since the car's front had crumpled. Her head flopped like a rag doll. There was blood everywhere. The passenger-side door could be opened, and the girl there was covered with blood but was breathing and half-conscious. Bystanders managed to help her out of her seat, freeing up access to the driver who was motionless and apparently dead.

I jumped into the bucket-seated car to try to reach the driver. She was not breathing. She had a large head injury such that she was almost scalped at her forehead area, with a huge gash. So much blood had dripped into her nose and mouth that even if she had an airway, she couldn't have taken a breath. I had nothing, no tools, a few handkerchiefs offered by the neighbors. I could hear and feel them getting out the girls in back, while I knelt on the passenger seat full of broken glass, never feeling it, to try to establish an airway and start mouth-to-mouth resuscitation. Later, I realized I was so sad for this child that I was weeping, but was so covered with blood that no one would ever know.

I was in such an awkward and precarious position, leaning over at an untenable angle, that I thought my muscles would give out before I could be effective. I worried about her neck, but I had no choice but to reach as far as I could to pull her upper body into the car from where she was wedged against the tree. There was a thick piece of bark embedded in the side of her head. With no airway, her neck would never do her any good anyway, I reasoned in that split second.

After trying to wipe some blood from her face, which was badly cut up with multiple lacerations, all of which were bleeding, I managed to maneuver to where I could cup my right hand under her jaw, my left on her scalp, and attempt to give her a breath, meanwhile harboring the futile hope she would start breathing on her own. She didn't. As I steadied and gripped her jaw, it felt loose in my hand, like a disintegrating skeleton. I realized her jaw had been broken in more than one place, and was hanging by its muscles. Still, I steeled myself and put my mouth over her mouth and nose, feeling both revulsion and heroism in equal measure. By then I knew there was no point, but I had to do it.

By then, I was really shaking, partly from sustained unusual muscular activity, on my knees, leaning over deep bucket seats and the obstacles between them, and partly from the high drama and urgency. I fancied I could save her life, even while I knew she was too far-gone. I could hear the police and rescue there behind and around me. They were huge guys; I knew they'd never squeeze in there like I could. They could see the predicament instantly and called for the "jaws of life," which I heard loudly in my ears, as though on top of us, as they started to saw away the steel from the tree in order to free her.

The rescue team told me to continue to do what I could until they could get her out. They handed me some suction equipment, not easily maneuvered. A mask was impossible in that position. I managed to get one or two breaths into her but they were clearly ineffective. I could not feel a pulse, so I pounded her chest once or twice, then I put my ear to her chest and thought I could hear her heart beating. I gave her another breath, and just then, her body contorted and a huge amount of blood and vomit came up and out of her mouth, some of it into mine, as I tried vainly to get out of the way. The gruesomely bitter stomach contents mixed with the sweet, sickly taste of blood and I frantically spit it out, feeling totally out of control in my revulsion and despair. Time crawled in slow motion until the rescue crew got the steel cut to get her onto a proper stretcher and over to the hospital, which was less than a mile away.

Generalism and Mission

CHAPTER ONE

The "Know-It-Alls"—The Work of The Generalists

What we all know is that no one can know it all. Any of us are lucky if we know even a little of what there is to know and what we ought to know, no matter what job we have. But some of us are actually comfortable knowing that we must at least try to know it all because that is precisely what our jobs call for.

We will be talking about medicine—and about generalism in medicine; but it really goes for any field. It is the generalist who attempts to embrace and hold closely that great body of knowledge that is one's purview, which is all of medicine. Instead of becoming exhausted and demoralized by the shear volume and impossibility of the job, the generalist is actually exhilarated by it. One becomes "curioser and curioser"—to borrow from *Alice in Wonderland*—because one is in fact in a kind of Wonderland of inspiration and excitement.

One may come upon a new idea or item of knowledge, or one may take a fragment of an impression and transform it into a solid, substantial part of one's own understanding. Both offer equal opportunity for fascination, often thereby launching a brand new facet of unexplored territory, or creating a fresh aspect of an old concept.

The imbalance between the security of the known and the danger or excitement of the unknown makes some seek sameness, while others opt for change.

Hence we have those who become very good at doing the same thing over and over again, able to get around a subject and know everything in depth (in medicine we call them "specialists"). And on the other hand we have the generalists, who are "specialists in generalism" (in medicine this would include the family practitioners, the internists and the general pediatricians)—the ones who look for breadth, for change, for a broad range of experience, knowledge and pleasure.

CHAPTER TWO

The Mission of Medicine: Not Just a Job

The mission of medicine is to heal the sick. When cure is elusive, it is to relieve distress, and always to comfort.[1] All of us who became physicians had our reasons, but we had to have a genuine interest and ability in science, and an appreciation of people as individuals living in families and societies. We had to be willing to work hard to learn and to keep up with all we needed to know. The profession self-selects its members, usually according to personal proclivities, to the benefit of patients.[2] Those of us who go into technical specialties may have some penchant, those who become psychiatrists some insight.

We who embrace generalism, without attempting to limit ourselves with regard to age, gender, disease or setting of our patients have the most interesting time of all.[3] We have to remember and revel in this, because the eclectic nature of our specialty and our patients can become a detriment in terms of efficiency and economy of resources.[4] It is much easier to do one thing and do it well, again and again than to stand ready to do everything and anything. The consolation prize is we're never bored. Another plus is that we become the only "real" doctors, in that we can take an undifferentiated patient, and fulfil most of his/her needs, using other specialists as needed.

Generalists, themselves come in different forms. The terms, primary care and family practice, have been fused recently, due to pressures outside of medicine, both governmental and commercial. But, although there is overlap, the terms are different.

Family medicine implies a discipline and a philosophy whereby the generalist learns to look at individuals over their life spans and in the context of their families. It implies continuity of care over many years and many generations.[5] It is best embodied in the country doctor who lives permanently in a small town or village and cares for a limited population. He/she gets to know nearly all the people, often in and out of the office. But the same concept can apply in large cities, where one doctor stays in one location for many years, and carves out a population of patients whom he/she knows and follows.[6]

Ideally, this practitioner is a physician, with the breadth and depth of training sufficient to diagnose and treat not only common illnesses, but to figure out and discover uncommon presentations of common maladies, as well as to think of rarer diseases which are bound to occur among a given population of patients.[7] Managing overlapping and complex multiple illnesses present in a single patient is another skill not easily undertaken by ancillary personnel such as nurse practitioners and physicians' assistants attempting to do true "primary care." These functions are unlikely to lend themselves to protocols or algorithms. The ability to know when one does not know implies that one has at least known of the existence and pathology of the gamut of medicine, not just the likeliest presentations of illness.

Primary care, on the other hand, can mean the person first in line to see the patient. This person may or may not be a physician, nor need be trained in family medicine.[8] The type of care rendered say, to an acute sore throat, may be equal and equivalent according to protocol, for that single episode, but the Family Physician is able to pick up on other aspects of the patient's life, using the opportunity of the sore throat to get to the real meat of that person's future health as well.[9] For example, the obese, smoking patient whose strep throat is treated just fine, but whose real problems are ignored. Most of us, as part of our training understand that prevention is easier than cure (for those diseases that are preventable) and have incorporated the usual preventive measures into our practices. Some of us could do better at this function, with newer and better "systems" for locating and isolating patients likely to benefit, and arranging for group visits or other innovative teaching methods.[10] The truth is, that such tasks can be delegated to partially trained or even untrained people. Teachers in schools can take on the task of health education. With the Internet, given proper motivation, patients can educate themselves, although the COVID-19 pandemic has revealed, among other things, socioeconomic disparities that produce a lack of universal access to broadband internet access required for modern education

But it is the physician who catches that patient in the "teachable moment",[11] often when he/she is sick, and who realizes how illness can affect his/her life.[12]

More recently, physicians have been exhorted to have another mission besides healing the sick: to look at our patients as members of a population, and to think in terms of the outcomes of disease and death in the aggregate, as our public health colleagues have always done. One problem with that is that rare diseases can be overlooked, or even discounted. Some of us may think, probably rightly, that if we do an excellent job with each patient, the aggregate will take care of itself. As we master the more common illnesses we can afford the luxury of seeing well people before they become ill.[13] However, even in the most highly advanced societies, where public health outreach has convinced the population to live the healthiest of lives, still there will be sickness, and the need for the Family Physician to evaluate and to know when to intervene.[14]

No matter in what country one finds oneself there are problems.[15] For example, with more basic surroundings, one does not have to worry about being sued in court and one's life savings taken away. In the advanced countries, one is limited by turf battles and certification (other specialists may not want you doing procedures they feel is only their prerogative). If government or a commercial clinic is paying one's salary, it's too low. If one is in the marketplace vying for patients, one must worry whether patients can pay.

Some of us find ourselves practicing in settings not of our choosing, and not geared to make the most of our skills. Here, we have the most chance to prove our flexibility and our ability to "land on our feet." Of all the specialties, family medicine prepares us for various roles in the medical spectrum.[16] We have the opportunity to become the "most valuable player" on any medical/health team.[17] Having done more than one job in medicine prepares one for defining what role one really prefers, and one can progress toward one's goal as chance and circumstance dictate.

The important thing is to have the same sense of purpose that led us into medicine in the first place.[18] It is crucial to remember what a privilege it is just to know what we know, to understand the body and its illnesses as we do, and to be in a position to help our fellow-creatures in their worst distress. The day that any one of us wakes up to medicine as "just a job" will be a sad day in the life of an old and glorious profession.

Endnotes

1   Gordon, AS; End-of-life issues. Caring, 2001 Feb.;20(2):6-9.

2   Gorenflo, DW; Ruffin ,MT 4th; Sheets, KJ. A multivariate model for specialty preference by medical students. J Fam. Pract. 1994 Dec;39(6): 570-6.

3   Pruessner, HT; Hensel, WA; Rasco, TL. The Scientific Basis of Generalist Medicine. Acad. Med. 1992 Apr., '67(4): 232-5.

4   Rosenman, R; Friesner, D.; Scope and Scale Inefficiencies in Physician Practices. Health Econ. 2004; Feb. 24; 13(11): 1091-1116.

5   Mainous, AG 3rd; Goodwin, MA; Stange, KC. Patient-Physician Shared Experiences and Value Patients Place on Continuity of Care. Ann. Fam. Med. 2004; Sep-Oct; 2(5): 452-4.

6   Saultz, JW; Albedaiwi, W.; Interpersonal Continuity of Care and Patient Satisfaction: A Critical Review. Ann. Fam. Med. 2004; Sep-Oct; 2(5): 445-51.

7   Stephens, GG; The Intellectual Basis of Family Practice. J Fam. Pract. 1975 Dec; 2(6): 423-8.

8   Sidani, S, Irvine; D, DiCenso, A. Implementation of the Primary Care Nurse Practitioner Role in Ontario. Can. J Nurs Leadersh. 2000 Sep-Oct; 13(3): 13-9.

9   Whitcomb, ME, Cohen, JJ.; The Future of Primary Care Medicine. New Engl. J Med. 2004 Aug 12; 351(7): 710-2.

10   Solberg, LI; Brekke, ML; Kottke, TE; How Important Are Clinician and Nurse Attitudes to the Delivery of Clinical Preventive Services? J Fam Pract. 1997 May; 44(5): 451-61.

11   McBride, CM; Emmons, KM; Lipkus, IM; Understanding the Potential of Teachable Moments: The Case of Smoking Cessation. Health Educ. Res. 2003 Apr.; 18(2): 156-70.

12   Gorin, AA; Phelan, S; Hill, JO; Wing, RR. Medical Triggers are Associated with Better Short- and Long-Term Weight Loss Out-

comes. Prev Med. 2004; Sept.; 39(3): 612-6.

13   Flach, SD; McCoy, KD; Vaughn, TE; Ward, MM; Bootsmiller, BJ; Doebbeling, BN; Does Patient-Centered Care Improve Provision of Preventive Services? J Gen. Intern. Med. 2004 Oct; 19(10): 1019-26.

14   Stephens, GG; Amundson, LH; Bishop, FM; Bryan, TE; Burket, GE Jr; Carmichael, LP; Chisholm, RN; Ciriacy, EW; Curry, HB; Farley, ES Jr, et al. The Intellectual Basis of Family Medicine Revisited. Fam. Med. 1985 Sep-Oct; 17(5): 219-30.

15   Wainer, J.; Work of Female Rural Doctors. Aust. J Rural Health. 2004 Apr; 12(2): 49-53.

16   Fincher, RM.; The Road Less Traveled—Attracting Students to Primary Care. New Engl. J Med. 2004 Aug 12; 351(7): 630-2.

17   Qidwai, W; Saleheen, D; Saleem, S,; Andrades, M; Azam, SI.; Are our People Health Conscious? Results of a Patient Survey in Karachi, Pakistan. J Ayub Med. Coll., Abbottabad. 2003 Jan-Mar; 15(1): 10-3.

18   Spickard, A Jr; Gabbe, SG; Christensen, JF.; Mid-Career Burnout in Generalist and Specialist Physicians. JAMA; 2002, Sep 25; 288(12): 1447-50.

CHAPTER THREE

Doctors Doing Good: The Best Uses of Power

When I was in English class in high school—even then—there was the lament that we had lost our heroes. We were given a reprint of an article, I think it was from the *Saturday Review*, with the recounting of the history of heroes, and how we no longer have a sense of the heroic.

I disagreed then, and still do.

Every age and every point of view has its heroes—whether acclaimed or not, "sung or unsung." For what are heroes, but especially powerful, enviable and admirable examples to be held up for emulation by others? If everyone were to act this way, the world would be a better place, or I wish I could do what he/she has done.

In medicine, we have always had heroes; they walk among us, their ghosts inhabit our literature. Lately we've had quite a few antiheroes as well. The false heroism of those making more and more money, and taking more and more social power, becomes transparent.

Money has been the only possible vehicle for power and recognition for some; political office the only track for others. Trappings have prevailed over substance. "Perception is reality" became a popular phrase perpetrated on the gullible and the savvy alike.

Some of us physicians were persuaded to take antiheroes to heart, and to take their values as ours. What they think they need to give them power, we have never needed because we already have it.

Medicine, by its very nature, confers power, intrinsically. There is the power of knowledge—just the knowing, which gives the irreplaceable and pleasurable feeling of mastery. And there is the knowledge that—in a brisk blink, or a pensive hour—a diagnosis or treatment can be made which will completely change the life of another person. This is priceless power—even when organizations of hospitals, commerce and government attempts to control us unnecessarily, and to transfer rewards for using these powers to themselves. If we keep that power and declare the autonomy we should have (and have always had but are fast giving away to the highest bidders and the lowliest bureaucrats) we can maintain our own high standards, and reasonable return for our efforts.

Education and training cannot be taken away; the value and power of solid satisfaction, based in the reality of accomplishment, will always be more reward than its dollar-translation.

If we ever forget that, we will have lost the sense of our own daily hero-ism, which can't be bought.

CHAPTER FOUR

The Doctor You Want:
How To Get One and Why You Can't

All of us look for a doctor who will take care of our whole person, who will be available when we're sick, who will take care of us when we must be hospitalized, who will visit us in the nursing home when we're old, and who will also take care of our family members. Really, everyone wants that, even if they don't know they want it.

People today who have a complaint or symptom that's not an emergency almost have to make their own diagnosis to decide to which specialist they should go. (My knee hurts: do I see a rheumatologist or an orthopedist?)

Or they wait until they have something emergent, then go to an emergency room for that one thing, and go away thinking that, because they've had a zillion X-rays, scans and blood draws, that they've had enough medical care—that everything has been covered. But that's not the reality. Everything hasn't been covered. The greatest threat to your health might be something totally irrelevant to that particular episode. Worse, more might have been done than was needed, finding hidden "threats" that turn out, after more testing, to be nothing after all.

The Internet purveys as much misinformation as information, especially where medicine is concerned, since you can't tell the hype from the science, without having studied medicine, but having experienced the broad practice of medicine, as in the residency and practice of a generalist.

Those who have gone into a technical specialty right after medical school, are much admired and much sought after for the specific things that they do, which usually involve some sort of technology. Hence, the reimbursement for their services is very high, even though many of the procedures done have not been strictly necessary, not from any dishonesty but only because when you're a hammer, everything is a nail. When you're equipped to do a technical task, and especially if the decision to do it is made by the same person who does it, there is an inherent bias toward going ahead with it.

These technician-physicians are mostly excellent at what they do, compassionate and knowledgeable physicians, honest and forthright, many of them trying to do the right thing regarding over-utilization. But the public, due to marketing and fascination with new toys, begins to demand what to them looks like "quality," because of its up-to-date appearance of cutting edge competence. Sometimes outright fear mongering is used by those marketing these procedures.

These specialists are reimbursed highly for their work, whereas the generalist who figures out what you really need, who saves you from a painful or unnecessary work-up, who does a low-tech version of a test that yields the same information as the expensive high-tech version (ankle-brachial ratio for peripheral vascular disease comes to mind), who pulls together the disparate parts of your story not just today but over time, is barely paid enough to keep his/her office open to continue to give the care they know people need. The managed care companies purveyed deals with hospitals to take care of all their patients, whereby "hospitalists" are hired to admit patients whom they don't know at all, cutting off the personal physician from being able to afford to admit their own patients to the hospital, since they cannot be paid for their work. Thus, at your sickest, you'll see someone who never knew you when well, won't follow you when you're out, and might not care about you the way your personal physician does.

Many family physicians and general internists have closed their offices and gone to work, on a salary, for a hospital or other business entity. Then they must adhere to the rules set up by that entity, many of which rules have more to do with the business health of the entity than with excellent medical care of the patients. Now there are schemes such as P4P, the so-called pay for performance, by which bean counters tally up how many diabetics get certain recommended test results. They are counting what is easy to count, and calling that an equation for a measure of total "quality," when it is a small piece of the puzzle, and then giving a bonus for adhering to the plan.

They are promoting the same behavior from doctors as from teachers whose students must pass a certain test, and must "teach to the test," rather than dwell on the best medical care for the patient or the best education for the student.

Whatever medical "system" or non-system prevails, if the fully-educated, fully-functioning, independent family physician, general internist and general pediatrician are missing we as patients will be missing the kind of care we all want and need.

CHAPTER FIVE

Family Doctors Would Need to be Reinvented

Yesterday, and every day, in my office we had one or two patients we call our "Oldie Goldies." People who have been with us since 1971 when I opened my practice, so many years ago. People whose progress, medical and personal, I've shared, and who share mine. We know their parents, kids and cousins either because they call us in crisis, or they're our ongoing patients. And every day we see at least one, and sometimes more new patients, usually sent by friends, who say at the end of the visit: "I'm so glad I found you! I'm so sick of seeing specialists who don't really know or care about all these details and don't pull it all together."

Every day in my office I do some procedure which others might refer: punch biopsy, flexible sigmoidoscopy, ear lavage, endometrial biopsy, breast cyst aspiration, etc. Specialists do them with equal, not better skill. But my patient is served better (and cheaper) by me, because I also address other problems often in many organ systems, without restricting myself to the "code" of the visit's description.

Generalism in medicine is especially valuable now, with burgeoning and confusing information abounding on the Internet. Especially now, when the "baby-boomer generation" is aging: its women are entering menopause, its men are facing prostate risks. These savvy people want preemptive comprehensive knowledge and management from their physicians when well. They want judgment and careful diagnosis and choice of specialists when sick.

No one but the family doctor sees that as his/her role. The gynecologists are not that interested in heart disease, hypertension and diabetes and are not up on the drugs, except in their field. The general internists often don't do procedures and few want to get into gynecology, and the urologists have no interest in anything but plumbing, though they're very good at it.

Family doctors obsolete? Not on your life. Public wants specialists? You bet. So do we. When we/they need them. Not before.

The specialists are becoming increasingly narrow in their scope and abilities. The patients know this. It is proper and understandable as special procedures advance. An important position we could take is to advocate against enabling specialists to capitalize on their exalted positions, with our aiding and abetting, by hiring "physician extenders" whose scope of practice exceeds the specialists' abilities to "supervise" them. I am referring to the vascular surgeon who hires a nurse practitioner to "cover" all the medical problems for his patients which he himself not only hasn't kept up with, but never knew in the first place (drugs for hypertension, diabetes, etc.). Or the cardiac surgeon who hires a Physician's Assistant (PA), allowing him to round on his patients, expecting him, for example, to pick up things like confusion resulting from overdose of lidocaine combined with hyponatremia, causing a patient to pull out a femoral line, which is beyond this PA's experience. Unfortunately, it may be other physicians and large groups who, for their own agendas, attempt to devalue the family doctor. Unless we oblige them and become triage officers, losing our knowledge and action edge, we do not have to comply with their judgments.

Some of us feel depressed when devalued by others and made to feel unneeded. Others of us know our value, and are proud of it. Our patients know it for sure, as long as we deliver that value in their service, which is our job.

This situation is relevant to the issue of hospitalists. It comes at a time when studies are cited charging multiple medication errors in hospitals. This is a time when countless pressures conspire to abolish careful and caring medicine. No matter which specialist admits a seriously ill or traumatized patient, or even a routine surgical patient, often there will be multisystem disease, much of it outside the specialist's field. Then either another specialist is called, who himself does not see his role as overseer of the whole patient, or nursing staff is depended upon to know and obtain a comprehensive view of the patient. Nurses are wonderful, but shifts change every eight hours. They can alert to ominous signs but are not trained to spot early emerging pathology based on vast knowledge of disease processes.

Rather than removing the family doctors from the hospital or proclaiming their obsolescence, they should be utilized as the generalists needed to fill the bill, involving one in every hospital and icu case. Perhaps calling one in as consultant, if the patient did not have a family doctor before, but not attempting to displace him/her by someone who trains and stays only in hospital.

Nurses, even well-trained "extenders," are not physicians; specialists are not generalists. Two true statements which, when understood with their full implications, bolster the role of the family doctor, both in office and hospital.

Often I describe to patients the family doctor's role as the hub of a wheel, the spokes of which lead to specialists when needed, returning to the hub for ongoing care. If the family doctor were ever to be unwisely edged out of patient care, that would be one wheel that would need reinvention.

CHAPTER SIX

Continuity, Control and Gatekeepers

Until only recently, medical generalists were being seduced by large medical organizations with the lofty title of gatekeeper, after a period of having been virtual step-children of medicine, low men and women on the totem pole. There was a suggestion—made possible only by the elevated status of the bean counters—of retraining "specialists" to do "primary care," in new health plans, run by businesspersons or physicians-turned-business-persons. With a more recent pendulum swing, patients can see "specialists" ad lib, and costs have run completely amok. Generalists have been reduced to triage officers and no longer care for their sickest patients in hospitals. They are fast losing status and prestige, because those two imposters are hooked to money, and procedures in medicine are paid well, while careful, thoughtful diagnostic and management skills with continuity are not.

Even with healthy habits and perfect preventive care, eventually illness occurs. We need plenty of tertiary-care skilled specialists in excellent hospitals keeping up with the innovations of the day, to be able to choose the best care when our patients require special or intensive treatment.

Generalists have honed their skills in prevention, early detection, in sorting out undifferentiated disorders, and in managing both chronic and acute illness, choosing consultants when needed. They can give care with continuity to everyone.

But how is continuity possible when systems encourage "competition" leading to employers (not patients) changing plans yearly for the best deal? How many of our patients have come back to us, their long-trusted doctors, after being forced to try "plans," complaining they never got to see the same doctor twice, and the doctor they chose left or was dropped from the plan? If we join these plans, how can we sign their contracts, and still offer optimal care?

Basking in the glow of being recognized as "important" and as "gatekeepers" by commercial medical organizations should not have contributed to an enhanced self-image. Arrangements whose bottom-line includes capture and control of both patients and physicians, with regard to cash flow and medical activity, have proved not to be in the interests of either patients or physicians, or medicine as an independent profession.

Does this mean that we should eschew all organized medical care plans (HMOs) in which patients and doctors are captured and controlled? The best of such plans can provide adequate care, and many of us may choose to work in these plans, doing a creditable job. But we must not pretend that this is ideal, or an improved version of medical care, or even desirable regarding costs. A government study in 1994 stated that Medicare recipients will no longer be encouraged to join HMOs because HMOs do not save costs after all.

Who will defend and protect the rights of the great majority of people who wish to be free: doctors, to do what they know is best for the patient; and patients, to obtain for themselves medical care according to their own choices?

Who, then, are the real gatekeepers?

Who can argue with the laudable goals of universal access and coverage? But who wishes the demise of the independent doctor and patient in the process? How are freedom of choice, and continuity of care to be achieved at once? Right now?

Actually—rather simply. And not by either of the ascendant plans proposed in the past: neither the Clinton plan of 1994 (managed competition) nor the single-payer plan (Canadian style). And probably not by any new scheme of centralized planning extant among today's politicians, no matter how well-meaning. The backers of such plans often have their own agendas, tied to the power of the purse they wield and plan to control, and this includes even some of our own medical organizations. Any so-called plans that do not encourage freedom and choice, and are antithetical to continuity, such as employers able to change plans yearly, tying patients to their employment plans with changing lists of doctors, doom us to chaos, waste and abrogation of control over our own health and destiny.

Only the HSA (Health Savings Account) idea, now that the requisite change in tax laws give patients control and incentives, with or without employer option to participate, will accomplish both coverage and access, and will lower costs as well. This idea was proven by the Quaker Oats Company between 1983 to 1985. (*American Medical News*, January 3, 1994, p.39) Patients save money in tax-advantaged IRA-type accounts which roll over if unused yearly. High deductibles and community ratings assure affordable coverage for all. Over-utilization is a thing of the past since patients are spending their own money. The patients' *direct connection* with costs keep prices down as in any marketplace where freedom survives.

When opponents paternalistically doubt that people will spend their own money on their health, they do not figure in the powerful role of imaginative, motivational public health advertising. There must be concomitant enhancement of on-going, targeted public health publicity countrywide to make health a popular habit even among the poor. Certain items, such as immunizations, could be separately subsidized to assure maximal participation.

Certainly, the very poor and marginally poor will require government clinics. But the rest of us will be able to retain a good portion of what we now are spending unnecessarily on "insurance," and still be able to choose freely the medical care we prefer.

Who are the real gatekeepers?

Only nineteen to twenty-one percent of the entire medical costs "pie" represents fees from physicians; over half of that is overhead, leaving physicians pocketing ten cents of the entire pie. Who are the recipients of the other ninety cents? Many are organizations with their own bottom-line business agendas: insurance companies, hospitals, home care companies, and soon, newer bureaucracies variously labeled, all inflicting rules, codes and enterprises that soon outstrip in cost and talent the basic enterprise of medicine itself.

The true gatekeeper is the one who serves the patient, not an amorphous organization with its own agenda.

Most persons use a hospital for a tiny fraction of their lives—but everyone needs a doctor, year after year. Yet the true generalist physician is fast disappearing, because of skewed incentives. Skilled anticipatory preventive care will preclude needing the hospital, since illnesses will not become critical as often. "Vertical integration" is a device by which hospitals, plans, bureaucracies and other so-called medical organizations try to trap every medical transaction between doctor and patient, claiming part of the action. Organizations have no automatic right to exist: the only real mandate for existence belongs to patients and those with the expertise to make and keep them well.

If anything should be captured and controlled it should be expensive, inflated costs of hospital care (one-fourth of which is administration), durable and disposable medical equipment, ancillary labor, insurance (both health and malpractice), legal fees, regulatory activity and many other over-priced items, not individual physicians and patients.

Who are the real gatekeepers?

Generalists have always been keepers of the gateway to patients' access to other expertise, but in the interests and employ of our patients. We take the time to analyze, diagnose and manage their many interrelated problems, both medical and psychosocial. We help them by suggesting referral only when needed, managing care persuasively, not dictatorially. As true gatekeepers, in the service of our patients, we can stand proudly.

But assuming paternalistic roles for organizations with which we have signed contracts separates us from our patients—even if "we physicians" have become the executives and are controlling the organization.

The cruelest twist is that as primary caregivers, we have not in fact been so personally advantaged as many have long assumed. We are back to being low men/women on the totem pole. Our valuable role is being devalued. We have abdicated our sickest patients (because the "plans" won't pay us for the continuity required in the hospital). We are being replaced with "physician-extenders," so that global budgets (another disastrous idea) can be met. These substitute generalists/gatekeepers will have the appearance of doing the same job, but will not have the in-depth background required for the most complex job in medicine, caring for the whole patient lifelong.

Who are the real gatekeepers?

All of us can become real gatekeepers—patients and physicians alike. Patients, with Health Savings Accounts (HSAS), will control their own money instead of enriching insurance companies. They will wisely control their own medical utilization, with insurance back-up for large bills. Physicians will keep open the gates to the best medical judgment based on bonds with patients, unhampered by other contracts. We will not break faith with our duty to each patient. We will hope that reality, morality and real medical care with continuity creep back into today's distorted medical world.

CHAPTER SEVEN

Breaking up Medicine While Claiming to Integrate it

There is a pervasive mismatch, getting worse, between medicine's stated mission to view the big picture and treat the whole patient, versus the perceived need to break that picture into pieces to arrive at scientific truth, medical necessity and cost-effectiveness.

The art is giving way to the perceived elements of science upon which it presumably is based and, in that very yielding, is losing some of the science and all of the art.

All the while continuing to cite the need for treating the patient as a person, and forging a meaningful doctor-patient relationship. All the while citing studies showing that the immune response is colored by the confidence and social condition of the patient. (Survival in breast cancer improved by support group attendance.)

How else to explain how we break the seamless "complete physical exam" into "screening procedures" according to sex and age, then attempt to do those and only those with double-blind, placebo-controlled proof of "medical necessity?"

Even in a patient with no stated symptoms, a complete physical exam can uncover disease, will cover all screening needed in that patient, and allows for assessment over time when done by the same physician. It is during that process of history-taking that a physician forges a bonding and trust with a patient, and gets to know myriad nuances, not just facts, many of which don't translate into a checklist.

The value of this relationship can be measured in lack of unnecessary emergency-room visits in the middle of the night, when a phone call to someone skilled and available who knows you will suffice. It seems almost ludicrous to verbalize these advantages, but so many in our bureaucracies and "scientific" establishment seem to have forgotten them.

The vexing evolution of "coding" and "medically necessary" activities, which have become an end in themselves, spawning expensive and medically unnecessary whole businesses, is an outgrowth of this dissonant and invalid thinking. What originally was a means for medicine to advance, by identifying definite diseases and studying them, has become a charade of labels, half of which are not even valid, since—as often as not—we don't know what the patient has until we test for it. But we're not supposed to test for it without the "diagnosis."

The idea of generalism has always been a valid one, since the family doctor has always stood for the melding of body and soul in the setting of people's real lives, in sickness and in health. But the new movement toward "primary care," being a child of cost-cutting, is actually a negation of that impulse to bring it all together, to encompass all the patient's needs.

Rather, it arrives as a half-baked mandate, a frantic impulse to provide something that will be more than nothing but cost the very least possible under the terms of their contract and coverage. The patients can tell in a minute what they're getting and not getting.

Large, randomized studies are necessary to solve basic science problems of whether one drug or procedure works for a given condition. Even these studies, however, do not always come up with the "right" answer (witness the differing conclusions of comparable studies). These are tools for a fully-educated, experienced physician to make shared decisions with his/her patient.

This data should not be misconstrued as final facts to be plugged into algorithms, which always make sense regardless of the individuals or the settings in which they are treated.

Example: All the studies showed that giving 0.3 milligram of estrogen was insufficient for osteoporosis prevention. However, some of us, realizing that some women have their own estrogen and don't need the full amount in pills, and that others simply can't tolerate the full amount, being limited by breast tenderness, etc., have—for years—been giving a half-dose in the appropriate setting, believing that some was better than none. Now comes the study that validates that course of action: a half-dose does prevent bone loss.

Certainty is nice, but medicine is practiced always in a milieu of partial knowledge and emotional intensity. The splitters are gaining ground over the lumpers, to the detriment of the patients and the profession. Soon, the art of medicine will be gone with the wind, broken into pieces, while at the same time lip service is given to returning to "primary care."

CHAPTER EIGHT

Second Opinion: Generalist Physicians— Added Value in a Crisis

Generalist physicians have the hearts and hands for helping in emergencies. Whether volunteering in droves for the challenging and unpredictable tasks that disasters breed, like those of Hurricane Katrina (as evinced by comments culled from the American Academy of Family Physicians (AAFP) Website, or acting as good samaritans in the public arena, they are prepared.

Starting with a foundation of broad, well-rounded education and training, the generalist grows in confidence by learning to deal with uncertainty and the unexpected. While ongoing education, journal reading, and "keeping up" are a way of life for all good physicians, generalists are attentive to continuing their in-breadth attitude and approach, and these are the qualities that make them so useful in unpredictable crises. That's what it takes to manage a makeshift clinic in an emergent situation in which anything can—and often does—happen.

The habit of humility, fostered by knowing that there's a subspecialist for every malady, informs the choices of generalist physicians and helps them know when it's time to call for assistance. The hallmarks of the generalist are the ability to see the big picture, the refusal to specialize narrowly, and the broad acceptance of whatever patients or medical problems may present for care.

At a time when aspirations to practice family or internal medicine seem to be waning among young physicians, partly because of perceived lack of "value" (like better pay or working conditions), we suggest they heed the lessons of realities versus perceptions. All our patients—not just the ones we'll treat in disasters—want an all-around doctor to take care of them, to know what to do for most of their ills, and to have remedies at the ready. In other words, they want us to be specialists in their comprehensive and continuing care. Added value lends added satisfaction to the generalist's lifelong professional and personal contentment.

CHAPTER NINE

What is a Good Doctor
and How Do We Make One?

Our patients—not we—are the ones to answer the question, "What is a good doctor?" Their verdict rings clear every day in the clinics and hospitals. They vote with their feet, their loyalty, their love, and even their willingness to heal. We receive that magnetic transmission and become better doctors because of their faith in us. Our trust in our patients fuels intellectual and compassionate energies toward a lovely, symmetrical synergy that is healing and inspirational.

Good doctors are born, not made. Just as Michelangelo understood the relationship of his choice of marble to his final sculpture, so we must realize that the good doctors are cooing in their cribs now, waiting to be delivered to the bedside, only molded, not made by us. Michelangelo believed that in every stark block of pure white marble a sculpted figure was trapped, waiting to be released. He trekked far to the Carrara Mountains to select and transport tenderly his chosen piece. Without talent and work the David and the *Pieta* would have remained trapped in the marble, just as without nurture and modeling, our gifted physicians will not burst forth.

At birth, good doctors are endowed with superior capacity for memory, not just for science and facts retained, ready to think about the ramifications of a complex case, but to remember names and faces they've seen, nuances day to day, management modifications, resources in communities, and where to look these up should their innate memory-talent fail them. They are blessed with superior reasoning ability to put together pieces of the puzzles of diagnosis and treatment. They are capable of emotional intelligence: the ability to gauge another human's feelings. They are gifted with temperamental qualities that are often oppositional, yet melded in one individual: patience with efficiency, strength with compassion, dispassion with warmth, toughness with love.

We must find these special people and make them our doctors. We can fill their empty slate. We have tried in good faith to do this through our schooling and entry procedures, but have probably failed at least as often as we have succeeded. Picking only compassionate people, or only highly intelligent or prepared people will not do: they will not have the other qualities.

As Rumpelstiltskin scoured the countryside until he discovered the spinner who could turn flax into gold, so must we magically mine our human quarries to uncover the good doctors lurking in the children of tomorrow.

CHAPTER TEN

The Rock Of Gilberto

There's one in Every Family: The Guardian
Gene and How it Holds us Together

Traveling the byways of medicine is an adventure into the human spirit, not just individually, but collectively. By that I mean small "collections" of people: families, couples, groups. All physicians see family dynamics unfold before them, if they're alert to the mini-dramas.

Family physicians, and those who assume that function yet trained in other fields, are privileged to witness heroic, yet deceptively mundane discharges of duty and performances of ongoing responsibility.

Everyone recognizes these special people. They themselves know who they are. There's one in every family, occasionally more than one. And if there is not, the family falls apart. They may embrace willingly their role, or kicking and screaming resentfully perform their assigned and unassigned task, but do it they will. They may weaken in their resolve, and often the burnout seen with such persons is identified as depression, chronic fatigue, and somatic symptoms.

What is it about these people? How are they different? Are they saints? Supremely talented, forbearing and confident? Or are they sinners? Moved by guilt to right some self-perceived wrong? Are they enablers? Doing for those who could have grown stronger doing for themselves? Are they losers? So insecure that they must constantly prove how dutiful they are? Does need for approval drive their conscience? Are their acts noticed? Or are the few deeds observed a drop in a pool of accomplishments?

What is it, really, that drives these people? Is this seen only in humans? Or do we see this phenomenon among animals within their groupings? We are not describing leadership, here. This is different, with only some of the features of leadership. This is taking up and accomplishing the undone, unwanted, individual and necessary functions shunned by others. Is the driving factor something different for each individual, each situation? Or is there a common thread? Could there be a "guardian gene" that predisposes certain individuals to take charge, to swim rather than drown? And to carry the tide of necessity with them, supporting and throwing constant life preservers to others?

These questions and their answers may be slightly different for each constellation of creatures we look at. Every family has its quirks. But the common thread through each is the existence of the "Rock of Gilberto."

One day my husband brought home a puppy. No warning. A large, black puppy, just weaned. It was the largest puppy that age I had ever seen. He said it was a pure cross between a malamute and a labrador. It belonged to his friend who fished with him on a boat called the Gilberto. We knew boats named for dogs, but never a dog named for a boat. Nevertheless, the puppy was instantly, obviously named Gilberto. We had three small children, I had just opened my medical practice, my husband's job called for him to be away a lot, and I just stared at this adorable puppy, realizing in a blink who would end up taking care of him, despite the protestations of husband and all the kids that they would. (This will ring all kinds of bells with mothers everywhere).

This darling puppy immediately claimed all our hearts, including mine, but this was a dog that grew while you watched. We said good night, and in the morning he was noticeably bigger. We relegated him to the back yard and soon, the entire yard was torn up. He jumped the fences and had to be put on a long run, which we devised.

One day, I was particularly harried, trying to juggle all roles, and my husband came back from out of town. I lit into him about how it was becoming impossible, and sputtered, "What do you think I am? The Rock of G—G—Ggg," trying to say "The Rock of Gibraltar." What came out was, "What do you think I am, the Rock of Gilberto?"

We both burst out laughing. From then on, in our family—and later for all my patients who heard this story, usually when I praised and encouraged them for being the Rock of Gilberto in their families—the emblem of carrying the load became the Rock of Gilberto.

That beloved, burdensome dog is long gone, but the symbol remains.

One of the families in my practice of thirty-two years has a huge range of problems. I explain to preceptees who rotate through my office (medical students or residents) that they can learn all of family medicine on this family alone. I have taken care of four generations over the past thirty years. There are at least fifteen members for whom I have had direct care, and many others who wander in and out from out of town. Here in Florida, we call them snowbirds, since everyone wants to come here in the winter. Some even have required care long-distance by phone. The mother (now grandmother and great-grandmother) has been the Rock of Gilberto, shouldering all manner of physical and mental illness burdens among her children, husband and grandchildren. The picture is never static. New diseases and situations are always cropping up suddenly. One of her daughters is assuming the role in the next generation, and one of the grandchildren in the next. It's a beautiful thing to watch: the glue that holds this family together. Most of my role as physician, apart from treating each person's own laundry list of diseases is just knowing and watching this happen, and letting the mother know how important and valuable she is. I think she already knows. When I discuss it with her, as a phenomenon, including her function and responsibilities, she cannot even imagine how it could play any other way, or what life would be like otherwise. Yet in other families from my vantage point as their physician it is easy to see how others feel the heaviness, and drop the ball that she carries so well.

My father was the "Rock of Gilberto" for his family, and his mother for hers. She was a Hungarian immigrant who came over in the bottom of the boat ("steerage") at fifteen years of age, and eventually, single-handedly through persistence and hard work, brought her parents and six siblings from Hungary. My father was the one who helped all his aunts, uncles and cousins whenever they needed it. My father and grandmother were the unsung heroes of their generations, and no one ever knew it, except those close to them.

Paradoxically, understandably, the ones most helped were often least grateful. Both father and grandmother took it in stride, without bitterness, but with certain chagrin. They never learned the lesson that they should stop. I never knew why they and not others in the family took on those roles. One qualifies, not in advance, but after the fact.

It carries no title, no fame, and no reward. It is what it is and we can't visualize otherwise.

It looks like I get the duty now, and I myself don't understand why, which accounts for my interest in the phenomenon.

I hope some research sociologists will be inspired to look at it. There has been research into altruism, and its qualities, but this is a different phenomenon. The genetics of this Gilberto guardian gene should be fertile fodder for the new generation of genome geniuses. I'm beginning to think that—like shyness, which we now know is genetic—this "Rock of Gilberto" characteristic is inborn, ingrained, and inevitable for the individuals that inherit it. We can't even take "credit" or blame for it.

There's one in every family, probably evolved for our protection and the maintenance of family units as viable, sustainable and cohesive vehicles for our success as a species. For now, that'll have to be good enough for me.

Patient Stories

CHAPTER ELEVEN

The Heart of Family Practice

The startling realization that the young nurse was acutely suicidal dazzled us both. She saw no way out. She planned to drive her car off a bridge.

She had approached me in the hospital.

"Could I come to your office? I haven't felt well." The visit yielded vague symptoms. She looked distressed.

A deluge of tragic emotion tumbled out. She supported herself and six-year-old child, she had a restraining order on her abusive husband, she filed for divorce, her father died, her mother was no help.

She refused group or psychiatric referral citing lack of time and money. She couldn't pay me. She barely got herself to work and her child to school.

I begged her to see a psychiatrist. She insisted it would blemish her "record" and jeopardize her job.

Despite my hectic day, I had to take time and think of a strategy. I couldn't betray her trust using involuntary solutions, as long as she could stay safe.

"Can you promise me you will do nothing to harm yourself for the next twenty-four hours?" I asked.

"Yes," she said, wracked with tears.

"Will you take some medicine?" She promised. "You need to call daily by 2:00 PM—or I will call you. You will see me and get medicine every three days. That will be our plan." I told her not to pay; it could wait. I chose an antidepressant.

Within a week she began to eat and sleep. By two weeks she wanted to live. She began to lose her frantic look. She smiled.

Within six months her depression lifted. After four years, she remarried, and the office received payments.

My real payment came the moment she first smiled, and gains interest whenever I see her in the hospital where we both still work, twenty-five years later.

CHAPTER TWELVE

I Sang With My Patient

She smiled fetchingly and threw her arms around me. She was so happy to have someone to hug. She was large, obese, kyphotic and almost bent double while edging slowly with her walker toward the examining room. She had sent a Christmas card and a birthday card, and I thanked her for them, while secretly praising myself for remembering she had sent them.

She was diabetic and hypertensive and eighty-eight years old, and had just stopped driving altogether, having made a judgment of her own that it probably wasn't safe. She had all her marbles. It was her son who took care of her, both of them all that was left of a family, but he was as immobile as she was, already elderly himself and in need of bilateral hip replacements.

Her blood pressure was too high, though her diabetes was in fair control, and she said, "Well I'm on so much medicine, and it's still high, so I guess it's just going to be high all my life —and I am eighty-eight, you know."

I thought about all the bean-counting going on these days, and how "quality" is being judged, by what's easy to count. Many of us physicians wonder, from examples in our daily practice, if maybe most of the real quality in the "doctoring" we do isn't subject to numerical measurement.

As I questioned her in minute detail, after I noted foot and ankle edema, and quite a few pills left in her diuretic bottles, it turned out that she would never take the diuretics when she planned to "go out," meaning leaving the house for any reason, which was often. And when she returned to the house, she didn't take them either. And at night she didn't take them because she didn't want to be up urinating. We had had this conversation before; with me trying to impress on her that if she peed it was because she needed to, to reduce her blood volume and thus her pressure. She did get the connection, but she didn't care to make the effort, yet she always denied depression, and would never accept medication or non-drug methods offered for depression. She admitted to cooking with salt like she always did—indeed, to liking salt—*a lot*, and to not paying any attention to what she knew she should be doing. She was vying for the title of my nicest, but most non-adherent patient.

I asked about her activities: she used to sing in the church choir, and since I also sing in a civic choir, I was interested. Last year I had noticed some fresh energy and new vigor in her demeanor, her dress, her affect. When I asked her why she was so upbeat, she had mentioned, blushing, that the young man who ran the choir had complimented her several times, and that she thoroughly enjoyed her rehearsals and her interaction with the organization. I could see that she had become quite enamored of this young man, and at one point, even began to believe that he had some feelings for her. Then one day, she came in, dejected, and trying to hide it. But I knew her well by then and could tell something was up. She came clean, with tears in her eyes.

"He's leaving, and I feel just awful." She couldn't believe he could just leave when he had—in her mind—become so close to her. She told me that—no—she wasn't interested in singing in the choir any more.

She said she had bought herself a harmonica and was learning to play it, and she brought out a small harmonica and began to pump air into it, attempting a tune.

"Oh, yes," I said. "What my father used to try to play. He made a good effort. He used to love one song especially."

"What was that?" she wanted to know.

"You'll probably know it," I said, "though none of the younger people would. It's 'There's a long, long trail a'winding....into the land of my dreams.'" I started singing the first line, not intending to give a concert —but she took it up, and in a second, neither one of us could stop, each filling in the gaps of memory of the words to that ancient, plaintive ballad, until the last wistful line, perfect for harmonizing, and then hanging on the final steady, perfect third—in true barber-shop style. Our eyes met, in a communication that can only be had through music. We laughed like schoolgirls, and hoped the rest of the office hadn't been listening through the walls.

This time, when I asked her if she could make the effort to comply with what we both knew was good for her, she actually said, "Yes—I'm really going to try this time." As she left the office, she said, "Maybe I should go back to the choir."

"Yes," I said. "Maybe you should."

CHAPTER THIRTEEN

Balance, Timing, Proportion—Best-Laid Plans and Bad Burns

Our own attempts to balance our lives, between duty and diversion—between family and work, work and play, play and creativity, creativity and reflection—are really attempts to organize meaning and significance out of an experience of life—the practice of medicine—that could and has become for many, an all-consuming passion in an unhealthy way. There are data to show that every year an entire class of medical doctors is lost to suicide. Physician burnout is a real phenomenon. That the profession self-selects troubled and depressed people may be a cause and/or a consideration, but is a hypothesis as yet untested. Even if true, it would require even more attention to the problem, with the development of a few "public health" measures to combat it.

Although the physical maladies of our patients vary greatly, one theme runs through all patient encounters: the meaning of the illness (or health) to individuals, and the part played by stress, tension and worry in their lives. We spend much of our time encouraging restoration of balance, good timing and a sense of proportion in their daily lives. We are taught to pick up on clues to their depression and anxiety, and to diagnose and treat these when non-drug methods do not work.

Yet often, we are not consciously caring for the most important person in the equation: ourselves, without whose health—mental, emotional and physical—we can help no one.

For my own play, diversion and creativity, and to balance my own life, I chose mainly music, and always looked for a community or university chorus in which to sing, no matter in which city I lived or how busy I was.

But one never knows how closely one's diversion and one's duty may converge.

I was singing in the University-Civic Chorale in Miami, whose conductor is an icon in choral music nationally and internationally, and whose wife is a well-known local artist and a patient of mine. One of her unique specialties was making paper, which entailed handling huge vats of boiling materials.

One Tuesday night, from 7:30-9:30 PM as was my wont, I was happily singing, after a full day's work. The singing itself is work, but different. One needs to stand most of the two hours, and concentrate on reading and perfecting the music. The loyalty is always to the music, over any personal concerns.

My beeper (before cell phones) went off at around 8:45 PM. Usually it's something I can handle from my phone in a few minutes, before resuming the rehearsal. I gathered my purse, chorus folder with music, and went outside the choral room to call. This time it was the emergency room of my hospital, and the patient was the choral director's wife! From the ER doctor, I got that she had burned herself pretty badly but was alert, awake and basically okay, at that moment.

My hospital was only two miles from the rehearsal, so I was faced with one of those decisions that one hates to make, for fear of choosing—of two simple paths—the wrong one. I agonized only a minute before deciding to let him finish out his rehearsal without interruption, while I went to the ER to assess the damage. I scribbled a note to the graduate student assistant of the chorus to be sure to give to him immediately that the rehearsal stopped, and I took off for the ER.

A.J.'s story was that she was carrying a huge vat of boiling material for her paper-making, when she tripped and fell, pitching forward while the liquid heaved backward, and felt the mass fall over her back, buttocks, back of her legs, shoulders and arms. The mass was of paper pulp, etc., and heavy, so that once soaked into her clothing, it stayed, absorbed and burned severely, at a temperature higher than boiling. She was in excruciating pain, some of the lesions were full-thickness, and it was obvious that the Burn Unit down at Jackson Memorial Hospital was where she would be headed.

This was a burn that could threaten life, both immediately, short term and long-term. This was a burn that would induce painful scarring no matter how skillful the rehabilitation. I was shocked, sad and very much involved, in such an ironic way.

I did not know if my director or my patient, his wife, would be furious at me for letting him finish the few minutes of his rehearsal, but he was so happy and lost in the music, accomplishing with his/our chorus the perfection and attention to detail which was so important to him and to us, that I couldn't see how allowing a clean conclusion to the rehearsal would make any difference where his knowledge of his wife's condition was concerned, since he wasn't the determinant of her well-being at that point.

No, I decided again—by now it's 9:15 pm— but to bolster my confidence I get A.J.'s opinion.

"How are you feeling—apart from the pain of the burns?" I asked her.

"Oh, don't worry about me. I'm fine," she said bravely.

"A.—I was beeped out of rehearsal. I left a note for your husband for as soon as it's over. Should I have interrupted him to come right now? Shall I call the choral office right now?"

She smiled through her pain.

"Let him finish the rehearsal—it's just a few minutes, and he has so few rehearsals in which to prepare the chorus."

I went to work, along with the doctors in the ER, to stabilize her (she also had high blood pressure, and was on medication for that), and detect any possible antecedent to the fall. Her husband showed up within the next thirty minutes, having been duly told to come directly to the ER, but that his wife was doing fine for now.

When I saw him, he was too concerned to be struck by the coincidence and the irony, or to be upset with me, since he figured I really didn't know the extent of it, which was true.

After explaining to him, but not yet to her, in detail (but as gently as I could within the bounds of truth and my ability to predict), what the next few months would bring in terms of pain, risk and scarring, I got him calmed down at least to where he felt he had a handle on what he needed to know, what he could control, what to expect.

Then, I went about the administrative nightmare of getting her into the burn unit promptly. That accomplished, a few hours later, I went home with the chords of the beautiful music I had been singing ringing emptily in my heavy heart.

Only much later did I realize, selfishly, how the episode had intruded upon my own need to gain some balance, some space, some peace. At first, when I pondered this irony of best-laid plans I was suffused with self-pity. In a flash, it was replaced by my solid satisfaction that these worthy people, whom I was privileged to know, had allowed me into their lives with one more privilege: that of helping them in a time of dire need. That revelation, which came as a bolt, gave me all the balance, timing and proportion I needed.

CHAPTER FOURTEEN

Pea Soup

I was pursuing my normal life, making dinner for my family. I was making pea soup, which I loved before its binding, grisly association with J.I., and even after. How else but by an uncanny ability to compartmentalize could I ever make pea soup or eat it again? Despite an active life in medicine, with often heart-wrenching cases, each of us physicians has another life just as other people do. Physicians grow up early in medicine, from the first day in gross anatomy lab, learning how to compartmentalize their minds and hearts so that they can take and take in what comes their way.

While stirring the soup the case of J.I. sprang unbidden into my memory, and I might just as well have been in the OR (operating room) of our hospital, looking over the shoulder of the surgeon who closed her perforated stomach and bowels that had been pierced by the bullet that shattered her spine, rendering her paraplegic. She had eaten pea soup that evening.

I got the call from Judy before she lost consciousness. I heard gasping.

"Dr. G. I've been shot! My husband—he's dead; he did it."

Then a child took the phone, crying hysterically.

"My Mommy's on the floor, she's bleeding. My Daddy's on the floor. He's dead. He shot her; he shot himself in the head." My mind was racing. I could hardly believe this scenario. I knew she had two little girls and that her marriage had been difficult lately, but I had not met the children or the husband, because of his reticence, and I was not clear on their ages.

"Are you hurt?" I asked.

"No," she bawled.

"How old are you?" I asked.

"I'm six," she sputtered.

"Did your Mommy call 911?"

"Yes, yes," she said. "My Mommy's eyes look funny."

I said, "The rescue people should be there any minute. Do you know your address?"

"No," she bawled.

"What about your phone number?" She stopped bawling for a second,

"I know my phone number," she announced triumphantly, and gave it to me clearly.

"Is your sister okay?" I asked.

"She's okay, but she's screaming. She's only four," she said through her panic and tears. I could hear the child in the background. I felt so helpless, so horrified. This is anyone's worst fear—that a suicidal, depressed person will make good his threats, taking his grievances, real or imagined with him to his grave, doing maximal damage on the way.

That a man could cripple his wife and take his life in front of his two small children is stranger than fiction. Yet not only can it happen, it was happening to my patient, and to me. I couldn't understand why rescue hadn't arrived yet.

"Listen, you're a very brave girl," I said. "You are a big help to your Mommy. Rescue should come in a minute; I'll call you back. Go and put a small pillow under your Mommy's head. We'll fix her up in the hospital."

"Okay, okay," she whimpered.

I called the operator who traced the phone number in no time. I called 911. They zeroed in on the house and found the nightmare as described. Judy was unconscious from having lost so much blood. She was in shock from the blood loss and abdominal trauma, and despite support with fluids and blood, she could have died right then.

The surgeon I called was particularly qualified because he had been in Vietnam. He entered the room after scrubbing, hands wet and in the air, saying, "This looks just like Vietnam," and I understood that he knew what a siege we were in for. I, too, scrubbed up, to be of some use, as long as I was there, and held retractors. The exit wound of the bullet was messy, as they usually are. The entry had been at almost point blank range at her back, at the level of T12 (the 12th thoracic vertebra, which is just above the waist). On its way out it had wreaked havoc with her insides, perforating the stomach and several loops of bowel, injuring her kidney and spleen. To everyone's amazement a well-spring of thick sludge, a green liquid, surged from the abdomen, over the incision, onto the operating table. She had just eaten pea soup for dinner, and her stomach contents had dumped into her peritoneal cavity!

We could smell the pea soup with its original odor; we could see the bits of ham in it, and a few intact dried peas. We were equally saddened and revolted, but we plodded on with what was at hand. After suctioning up most of the pea soup, Dr. H.Q. located the points of perforation, determined how much of each organ could be salvaged, stopped any active bleeding, and proceeded to suture whatever could be repaired. Mercifully, her aorta had been missed. If not, she never would have made it this far— she would have died on the spot. In the recovery room it was touch and go.

She had every reason not to survive. But I had known her as a determined, beautiful young woman who had faced odds before. I knew Judy would hold on and demonstrate that famous "will to survive" that all of us have witnessed in our medical lifetimes. I waited until Judy came out of the anesthesia. She asked where her legs were. She looked at me with panicked eyes, and I knew she understood that she was paraplegic.

"He always said he'd shoot me in the knees or back," she said. "I never believed him." The aftermath, recovery and rehabilitation took not months but years. Judy eventually took back full care of her children, adapted her house for wheelchair access, worked full-time, and became a competing wheelchair athlete, with basketball her specialty. For more than five years, I could not eat pea soup. Then, after a while, I could again, even while remembering.

CHAPTER FIFTEEN

Grand Subjects—Small Dramas:
Providence or Evidence, or Both

I looked forward to the spontaneously arranged lunch with special anticipation. Rona, my former office manager and medical assistant, had come to town from Atlanta with her two daughters on their way to a diving trip on the reefs in the Florida Keys. My office staff and I planned to take them to lunch overlooking Biscayne Bay. It was a lovely day in summer. We carved a swatch of time out of a busy, overbooked day just before my vacation. We had not seen Rona and her children for several years.

Eleven years earlier Rona and Monica, my present office manager, had been pregnant together, delivering within six weeks of each other, forcing me to work my vacation around them. They were quite a pair: Rona nearly six feet tall, and Monica, four feet eleven inches, such that when they stood facing each other as happened sometimes in our small hallway, Rona's huge belly nested neatly over Monica's in an expectant yin/yang symbol.

Rona kept in touch partly because she and Monica were friends, and partly because she could never forget that without me, as she was fond of saying with a grin, her children would never have been born. I was the one who figured out how she could get pregnant after a full, u.s. Army-led, specialist infertility workup for herself and her husband had proved fruitless—after she had resigned herself to the fact that she would never conceive. Now Rona's daughters, ages thirteen and eleven, living in Atlanta, could barely remember their lives in Miami. Only the drama of Hurricane Andrew stuck in their minds, from when they were five and three years old, still giving them nightmares.

As we sat down to lunch, Katrina, her stunning thirteen-year-old blue-eyed, blonde-haired nymphet of a child, just blooming into puberty, was giving me a big hug. I was overcome with astonishment and pride in how lovely she and her sister Sarah were becoming. Rona shot me a knowing glance, watching my emotions well up as I gazed on them as if they were my own children. Hers was a look that said, 'Thank you, yet again.'

At the time Rona had come to work for me she had been a helicopter pilot in the u.s. Army and needed a job. She left the army because her first husband also flew, and there was no spot for them both in Miami. I had received her application from the Florida Employment Office and almost discarded it. Yet for some reason, I interviewed her. Apart from an obvious tobacco smell in the room I was impressed with her easy directness.

I told her, "I cannot have someone who smokes."

"How did you know?" she asked.

"It's pretty evident," I said.

"Oh, you can smell it," she said. "Oh. Sorry. But I would never smoke on the job."

"You don't understand," I said. "You couldn't even smoke in your private life, though I guess it's against regulations as condition for hiring. But if I can smell it, so can the patients. Part of your job as office team is to help people quit smoking, the most correctable cause of death. 'Do as I say, not as I do' doesn't work."

Instantly she rejoined, "Then I'll quit now—for good."

My look of amazement must have impressed her. She hastened to add, "I have asthma. I should never have been smoking anyway."

"Well, that's for sure" I said. "But you have no medical training whatsoever, is that right?"

"Well, yes," she said, "I mean no. No medical training. But I'm a quick learner, if you'll teach me."

Taking a chance on hiring Rona was one of the best things I ever did. She did quit smoking, on the spot. She not only was a quick learner, she became the best phlebotomist I ever had, and was excellent with the patients, the right combination of kindness, caring and firmness. In such a small office we needed cross-trained staff. She quickly learned the computer for our billing system. She took over the management of the office and converted our antiquated accounting and check writing system into a computerized one. I never let her give injections; for medico-legal reasons I preferred to have a certified medical assistant doing that task, but for everything else she was priceless. I was panicked when, after ten years working with me, her new husband got word that he had to transfer to Atlanta.

It was especially ironic, considering the story of her pregnancy thirteen years before, that we met for lunch that certain day, one of my half-days in my private office. It had been one of the days that I got into a recurring debate about the "new," so-called "evidence-based medicine" (EBM) with an especially vocal faculty member at the family medicine residency program where I have worked part-time for four years, in addition to my private practice.

Evidence-based medicine attempts to determine best medical practices for clinicians. It is the latest sortie in the struggle for credibility among medical opinion-makers. By way of explanation: all of us wish for a reliable source of data to inform decision-making. Most of us try our best to keep up with latest studies and guidelines, changing our hallowed practices when data warrants. Medicine has always been practiced (by thoughtful practitioners) in this way. But not always has reliable attention been paid to how the data has been collected, namely, the quality of the data; therefore, addressing quality and standing of evidence is a priority and a problem, one that "evidence-based" practice hopes to solve. Thus, the large, double-blind, placebo-controlled, randomized trial has taken center stage, purporting to be the most valid evidence by which to make individual clinical decisions.

What can be threatening to clinicians is that experienced physicians are questioned for not sticking to new guidelines. Often these guidelines are produced from newly minted large studies that are generalized to individuals without knowledge of their special circumstances, although teachers of EBM claim to agree that patients must be individualized. The concept that adherence to "best evidence" is everything, and that individual judgment and long experience counts for nothing, has gained ascendancy to the point where the concept of "experience" is ridiculed as anecdotal, and put in a list under the "old, unenlightened way" versus the "new, evidence-based way."

The list showing the "old way" medicine was practiced usually contains language such as, "old gray-haired doctors conferring in a hallway." The new list shows "statistically-proven randomized studies." There is usually a heartfelt disclaimer that this does not lead to "cookbook medicine," and yet it appears that the ability to operate from an algorithm (cookbook?) is exactly what is sought. Nowhere is it mentioned that the individual patient does not read the studies, and may not fit into the profile of the people recruited for the studies. Nor is it inferred what surely is implied: that all one must do to practice medicine is to look at studies and never look at patients. Indeed, the concept of physiologic principles and biologic plausibility is held up as one of the main sources of error in the "old way." Even the "evidence" that a thorough examination of patients should be undertaken, is touted as on shaky ground. One is required to trust results of any large study done in multicenters with convincing statistics. Only years later might questions arise as to how really were those results obtained in each of those centers? And who's to vouch for them? And how often do their answers conflict with reality? We wait and are surprised when another study comes along to refute them. Still, one must trust something, mustn't one? What especially young proponents of EBM—and those who are older bot not active clinicians—sometimes forget is that the "anecdotal experience" is not just of patient care but of living through several of these reversal cycles and not being unreasonably influenced by the latest "final answer."

The reason for the special irony at lunch that day was that my solution, indeed inspiration, as to why Rona could not get pregnant involved chiefly the "old way" of medicine: experience, observation of prior cases, logic, knowledge of anatomy, physiology, microbiology, deduction, imagination, educated hunches and of course, luck. I had wished for some high-quality "evidence"—but there was none. One might say that the afore-mentioned string of attributes constitutes evidence of a different type, more often than not characterizing the real practice of medicine in the real world. It is wonderful to add, when available, some well-sought and obtained, more-carefully proven evidence. Most of the time and for most problems we do not have that luxury.

Rona's dilemma was just such a one.

One day in the office, after the patients had left, Rona and Monica and I had been ventilating a bit among ourselves about the difficult patients of the day. I encouraged this as a way of deflecting any impatience by staff while patients were in office, saving it for later when they could discuss and unburden themselves. One such patient had been especially testy, and they were hard put to understand why. I mentioned that the woman was actually grieving over her struggles and inability to conceive. I cited some other women who had the same problem and for whom I was able to offer help so that they became pregnant. I stated that perhaps it was chance, but I doubted it, since they had been trying for years, and had been through the usual fertility workups, but nothing had worked. I added that the process was surprisingly simple, just either overlooked or not believed by the specialists responsible for such workups.

Rona looked troubled during this conversation, and later called me aside to tell me about her own problems. I did not know her as a patient, but only as an employee, and I had assumed, wrongly, that she and her husband were not interested in having children. She became very emotional as she recounted her doctors' genuine interest, their examinations, their tests and follow-up, all provided by the extensive facilities and fertility specialist consultants of the u.s. Army Medical Corps, before she had resigned. She had gone as far as laparoscopy. Everything had turned up negative, with no cause found, and nothing to be done. I asked her what she would like me to do.

"Whatever you did in those other cases," she said. "Maybe it applies to me, too."

"Well, maybe," I said, "but maybe not. I don't want to promise anything, or to raise false hopes."

"Don't worry," she said, "I've lost hope anyway, but I can't see the harm in trying."

The next day I examined Rona. Although she had not complained of a discharge, her cervix looked a little red, with a mucoid yellow-white material on it, which was rich in white blood cells on wet smear. The vaginal walls were clear of discharge, and the wet smear taken from there had only epithelial cells. I did a Pap smear which came back normal but with inflammation. The bimanual was normal. I examined her husband, did a prostate massage which was negative as was his history, and sent him to obtain a complete semen analysis, including analysis for white blood cells on microscopy, and if any white cells or bacteria seen to do a culture and sensitivity. It came back with 5-10 white blood cells per high power field and with a significant colony count on culture.

This had been the exact scenario with the others who were unable to conceive: a wife with an untreated, unrecognized cervicitis; a husband with semen showing low-level bacterial activity, likely a low-grade, unrecognized, chronic prostatitis. How could sperm find such a milieu hospitable?

I explained to them my theory, of which I had no proof, only logic and circumstantial evidence. I told them I was willing to treat them for the presumptive infections with broad-spectrum antibiotics designed to cover both aerobes and anaerobes, reasoning that where there was one type of microbe, there might be others with different characteristics. They understood and agreed to the treatment, knowing that if they had any type of drug reaction or side effect, we had a shared responsibility that we perhaps were treating phantoms, but that the potential benefit—if it worked—would outweigh any risk. I told them to use condoms during and after the treatment and to come in for repeat exams.

Many years later, quite recently, I came across a few published references in the obstetrics/gynecology literature about unrecognized cervicitis and prostatitis treatment restoring fertility to couples. There were no large randomized trials, of course. Some (most) clinical problems do not lend themselves to such trials, and often those that are attempted are studying multifactorial issues, trying to isolate individual factors, and losing the individual patient in the process.

I gave Rona and her husband two full weeks of doxycycline, 100 milligrams, one tablet, twice each day and metronidazole, 250 milligrams, one tablet, twice each day. They returned for reexamination just as the treatment was ending. The cervical discharge was gone, the semen had no white cells, and cultured negative. I told them to resume relations every three days and enjoy life. After two months, Rona was pregnant!

The news of Rona's pregnancy permeated our work. The jubilation was palpable every day in the office. Just when I suddenly, self-centeredly realized that I would be losing a valuable assistant, Monica also became pregnant with her second son! Having attuned and adjusted all my medical life around my own three children, I could not exactly expect these loyal workers to do less for their families. Yet they both worked diligently and competently until the time of each delivery. I closed the office, signed out to my coverage arrangement and took a vacation while their absences overlapped. Each chose to return to work within two weeks, and the office smoothly continued on track.

Now we were all together again at lunch, and the reminiscences flew back and forth, along with the catching up and projecting forth of the future. I stared unbelievingly at Katrina and Sarah, Rona's beautiful and unexpected daughters. Lady Luck or Lady Logic? This was either providence or evidence—or perhaps a little of both.

CHAPTER SIXTEEN

Only the Translation

Sweet fatigue and righteous exhaustion came to him as the dying came to her. They had both put in a full day.

He had given the orders. The emergency room (ER) staff, competent as usual, had carried them out. His hours on the phone before finally sending Mrs. V. to the ER were filled with family adjusting medicine, following instructions by phone, and attempting to make her comfortable.

The large mass in her lung had defied definition, lying dormant for six unbelievable years. Two attempts at directed needle biopsy had yielded a demoralizing pneumothorax requiring a painful chest tube, and she had flatly refused open biopsy.

She had thrived, untouched, until just six months ago when her unlovely secret opened its petals and blossomed forth, planting new seeds inside lungs and all over pleura, flowering like cotton in Georgia, fluffy and ominous.

It was midnight, after a hectic office day for him. Mrs. V. had gone home from the hospital after a brief admission, and only two days had elapsed before symptoms again became unmanageable at home.

She must have wondered if now it was time to die. He didn't think so—but he couldn't know. They told him the blood gas results: they weren't good. They told him she was agitated and wouldn't breathe through her nose, so they replaced the nasal oxygen with a Ventimask.

They were waiting to get the gases again, but she was constantly upset, despite attempts to sedate her.

He knew he would do nothing more when he got there; he knew he could easily see her in the morning. He arranged the admission by phone and started to settle down, but he couldn't imagine, even with family around, her calming down now. He could only see her wondering where was he? He began to think that only he would have the healing touch that she needed now. Not only did they have their history together, as with all the patients in a family practice—the minor and major meanderings of bodily ills and emotional scrapes through the years—but she knew how often she had been helped to come through smiling, and it was sheer faith that could calm her down now.

She had a living will in the chart. They had had the "death discussion" long before, when she thoroughly realized that the single mass maybe could be radiated, maybe could be excised, and she chose not to do it—she chose to have faith that it really wasn't malignant (after all, the attempted biopsies were negative—though they had impressed upon her that they were so because they were admittedly inadequate).

"I'm old, I've had a good life—it's time to go. What am I staying for anyway?"

But now it was time to die, and it seemed more like time to stay. She knew that he remembered all of those conversations. He knew that whatever her blood gases, the agitation was part of that dilemma: wanting to go and wanting to stay. But more than anything, wanting to trust.

He threw on his clothes and went in. He couldn't do otherwise, even though he fought with himself, knowing tomorrow's patients in the office would be better off if he went to sleep now instead of going in.

He asked, who do you think you are? You know very well you're not indispensable—everything that can be done is being done. You know anyone else can do the job as well as you. Not only that, you know they could do it better, especially when it came to cure (after all it wouldn't have been you who would have removed that mass, had she allowed it). What if you were out of town?

But now it wasn't cure—it was comfort, it was solace. Was he being delusional? Or, in the middle of that self-deprecation did he have to be honest and recognize that only he would be the best comfort she could have. Could he deny her that? Now was when she needed it—not tomorrow morning.

So he went. As he walked in he could see her eyes. He had watched the respiratory rate from across the room, as he came in from the hallway of the Emergency Ward. He could see its striking change. He took her hand: she smiled weakly.

"Oh, I'm starting to feel better now, I think." Her son and daughter-in-law, to whom he had been speaking all night, and who did not expect him to appear on the scene changed their expression, and visibly relaxed.

"She's breathing a lot easier," they said.

The load, the responsibility, that he had been carrying all evening suddenly lifted, and he felt free.

As they looked at each other, his undying respect for the dying must have been revealed to her, as her silent message said, "I was waiting for my own doctor."

When he returned home, his wife, half-asleep asked, "How's your patient?"

"I think she's a little better," he said That was only the translation.

CHAPTER SEVENTEEN

Upon This Rock

She took my hand softly as I sat on the bed searching her face for clues—signals that would chart my way in this wilderness of feeling, this delicate kingdom of finely tuned communication. It was early Sunday morning.

"How difficult—how unfair it is—for it to fall upon you now," she said.

"I... I...," I began, not knowing at all what she meant.

But she continued.

"I mean to be the one to have to tell me." Her grip on my hand tightened and her eyes misted so slightly, then came clear again as I listened in reverent amazement. She continued, "...so soon after we've just met, I feel so bad for you— it must be very hard for you."

I returned her firmer grip fighting the desire to give way to the pathos of the scene with my own tears. I managed to smile a benign and, I hoped benevolent half-smile and said gently, "My only concern, of course, is you and that you know that there is treatment for this problem, treatment which sometimes works very, very well to control it—and that I will stay with you and take care of you in consultation with one of the most qualified hematologists we have on staff here."

I had a medical student doing a preceptorship with me at the time, and she had baked some brownies. She took that opportunity to offer them— and the spell was broken. Blessedly so. The mood became lighter and the physical examination for the morning progressed. I had just put Molly Lloyd in the hospital the previous day and when the tests came back I had had to tell her the truth, And here she was feeling sorry for me!

The resilience and courage of the human spirit are our privilege to witness, as physicians, nurses and other paramedical people, in ways that surpass any of Hemingway's novels with their often-contrived depictions of grace under pressure. Do we openly receive and appreciate these qualities and learn from them as perhaps we could? Do we realize how much more our patients know about certain things than we do? Do we realize how much there is to admire in our patients? If we fully appreciate them as people we probably do. Do we see how we are being repaid for our sometimes-extraordinary efforts with the opportunity of bearing witness to our patients' heroic examples? By their ability to face tribulations of often grand scales better perhaps than we could?

It seems so many of our doctor-written articles are condescending toward patients. We talk of our difficult patients, our "crocks" our "gorks." We never write of crocks formally, preferring to call them "difficult" patients. (For you, dear reader, who may happen not to be physician or nurse, a definition of "crock" is in order: it is many things to many people but its most convenient definition is probably, "A difficult, demanding and annoying patient whose problems are either mostly imagined or, if real, are made worse for himself and for everyone around him by his abrasive, whining or helpless personality.")

But we have never invented a word for the opposite of a crock. And tribute to the human spirit that it is, we see much more of that type of person. I might propose the term, "rock," to describe them and to call them.

Molly Lloyd was certainly one of those. She was a new patient. She had waited for me to come back from a short week's winter vacation instead of seeking medical attention elsewhere. She had formerly seen a surgeon who had done several needed operations on her, and a gynecologist for routine female "checkups" but she had no one to call if she got sick. She knew I was in family practice from friends of hers and she had intended to come in for a routine examination thinking she'd "try a woman doctor" for a change. But then she got sick.

She had sat in my consultation room for our initial meeting, recounting an ordinary enough story of what sounded exactly like the flu-like illness we were seeing a lot of that winter of 1977. She had fever, chills, severe malaise, nausea, some vomiting, severe myalgias, She was a devoted fifth grade teacher whose life was her work. Later I was to find out how much she would be missed. She stated that she had been so sick, that she even had to stay home from school the past two days. Yet to look at her one could not discern that she was acutely ill. She appeared bright, alert, and her conversation was smiling and pleasant.

To the end of the list of symptoms she had added, "'And lately I've noticed these funny blue spots on my legs—and all of my friends who had flu seemed to have gotten over the worst of it by a week or so, I've been wondering why I'm still sick."

"Well," I had said, "let's have a look at you in the examining room and we'll see what we can come up with."

One does not usually do a thorough and complete physical on every case of uncomplicated "flu syndrome," but my danger flags started flying when she mentioned spots on her legs, I had her undress completely so that I could assess the full extent of her skin involvement, and so I could palpate the size of her liver and spleen and check her lymph nodes. Sure enough, the "blue spots" were purpura and petechiae, she was pale, and had a fever of 101.6°. And her liver and spleen were enlarged. Even without blood work I was almost sure of the diagnosis but there was no way it could or should be even mentioned as a possibility without first confirming it for the shock would be unbearable, even and especially if it turned out not to be true, I tried not to let my face convey any alarm.

"Well, I can see that you've been really quite ill," I said. "You must feel pretty bad. You've been keeping a brave front haven't you? Trying not to appear as ill as you feel?"

Her shoulders slumped. "Well, Doctor, to tell you the truth I do feel pretty rotten."

I said slowly, "You know, there are a few things on your physical exam that lead me to think this may not be just a simple "flu" as so many others have had. We'll need a few tests to find out exactly what's going on, What I'd really like to do is admit you to the hospital."

"Oh, my goodness!" she said. "I don't want to go to the hospital!"

"Well, it really would be better," I said. "The nurses could observe you constantly and we'd be much better able to get the necessary tests and take care of you."

"When?" she asked.

"Now."

"Today?"

"Yes."

"When?"

"Now. Right now."

"Now?"

"Yes, it would be better." I spoke gently and directly, but quite definitely, without any ominous overtones.

She hesitated.

"Oh, Doctor," she said. "I so hate hospitals! I'd be so much more comfortable at home with all my own surroundings. Couldn't we do the tests from the office?"

I could see and feel her distress. Sometimes it does turn out that the patient didn't need to be hospitalized at all. That what they really had was a viral illness that would blow over with or without treatment and certainly without hospitalization. Our problem in medicine is that everything comes clear in the "retrospectoscope." With hindsight much can be asserted. But making decisions without all the facts is the art of medicine. And it is our lot to be required constantly to be definite when the real facts only allow us to be tentative.

"Of course, if you insist I must go right now, I will."

I hesitated, thinking that, if my worst fears were confirmed this might be the last time she would feel the warmth of her own home. I pushed the morbid thought from my mind, not knowing how prophetic it was, and told her, "Okay—today is Friday, The lab that I use will pick up soon today and do the preliminary blood tests overnight—they work all night to have results ready in the morning. If you definitely have to go in for further testing I'll call you tomorrow morning early." I knew that all I really needed was the CBC (complete blood count), at least to rule out or in my portentous working diagnosis. I also knew that a few hours one way or the other wouldn't make any difference at this point. I had my nurse write RUSH and, "call results to doctor," with my home phone number on the lab slip when she drew the blood.

At 11:00 PM the lab called. The technician was in a panic; the pathologist himself had been called in. "Your patient's white count is 69,000 with mostly lymphoblasts, 90%. The platelets are 80,000; the hemoglobin is 9.0. The pathologist came in special to check the slides himself."

"Oh my God," I said. "I was hoping it wasn't so, but I had suspected it."

"It's been double and triple checked," the technician said. "How old is the patient?"

"Only fifty-five," I answered flatly. "And it only happens to the nicest ones."

"I know," he said. "Isn't it always the way?"

"Not fair," I said.

"No," he said. "Not fair. I'm sorry to be the one to tell you, Doctor."

"I appreciate your calling me right away, thank you so much." I said bleakly.

He was another nameless face in the intricate network of human beings helping other human beings. Molly Lloyd would never meet him, never know how saddened this nameless face was by her misfortune. And he would never know what lay behind those blood cells on the microscopical slide.

I hung up the phone and sat perfectly still for a long time staring into space. All I could see was her face smiling through her pain and malaise. I had been struck by how pleasant a person she was—the kind of personality that seemed to have an innate serenity, as though incapable of hostility of any sort, without being sugar-sweet. Her appearance was neat, vigorous. Her hair was crisp, wavy salt and pepper combed back and full, She wore only a little makeup, and her slightly full tall figure was firm and belied her fifty-five years, Her face showed hardly a line and those that were there were smile lines. One would have said she was forty. I had first seen her as she walked confidently into the office. I had developed the custom in my office of always meeting new patients and getting their medical history in my consultation room before the patient was undressed, rather than putting them into the examining room directly. It gives a more equal footing to that initial impression which is so important to any relationship, especially the nebulous but unique doctor-patient one. The patient feels less defenseless, less regressed, less helpless.

So it was that I had first seen Molly Lloyd in my office. A medical student from Indiana was doing a one-week preceptorship in my office through the Department of Family Medicine at the medical school. She was with me when I had to tell Molly Lloyd that she had acute leukemia.

The medical student was an eager, bright, attractive young woman who was a senior, getting ready to make the decision as to the type of residency she wanted. It was this student who bore the pain with me when, in spite of unstinting efforts, qualified consultants and combination chemotherapy, Molly Lloyd died.

Often the drugs do give the longed-for remission (although adult leukemics do not as often have the typically good responses of children), but not this time. We kept her comfortable throughout all her suffering and when it was amply evident that all was lost, we did not add to the drama and the indignity of her death with last minute attempts to assuage any worries we as her physicians might have had that we had not "done everything."

We had in fact done everything and had lost. We did not insert extra tubes or attempt vain resuscitation.

Molly was given morphine for the pain of the extreme pelvic cellulitis she had developed which had preceded the septicemia and endotoxic shock which were the terminal events. She was also being given antibiotics specific for the organisms cultured from her blood, corticosteroids both for the leukemia and for shock, fluids and other usual supportive measures, Perhaps the morphine calmed her but she stayed conscious and saint-like, even whispering words of encouragement to us, to the very end, when her heart rate and respirations increased until she fell deeper into shock and simply ceased to breathe again.

The nurses in the intensive care units and from every floor where she had been were struck numb by her death, in spite of their usual closeness to fatal illness. She had rallied early in the course of treatment and we had all thought she would have a remission. We knew, of course, that the scene just played out would be inevitable some weeks or months hence but we tried to delay it some because that's what we've been taught and that's what we believe in. You never know when a tremendous breakthrough will be made—maybe in the two months between her remission and relapse? You never lose hope, even for miracles.

But as she was dying her best friend and room-mate who was an X-ray technology instructor with whom she owned her house had come to me and, fighting back tears, had said, "Please, Doctor, Molly and I talked it over several times in the past and we promised each other that we would not allow super-heroic, useless measures to be taken if all was hopeless. I don't want her to suffer—and above all I don't want her agony to be prolonged."

Barbara needed to feel that she had contributed something to the comfort and last wishes of her friends as indeed she had. Both Molly and Barbara were religious and their faith that this was Molly's "time" helped them through it all—gave it meaning. For them. To me, it was just another example of mankind coping with injustice.

I picked up the morning newspaper the day after she died. There were five different references to criminals, guilty of or charged with violent crime. None of them had or would have leukemia or any such deserved retribution. Only people like Molly—vibrant, contributing people who should live nine lives, not one cut short.

It was then, over my coffee, that my eleven-year-old son caught me with tears flowing unstoppable, down my face onto my newspaper, into my coffee cup. All the anguish, the living of those agonizing three weeks of fighting for her life—making critical decisions; calling the Blood Bank at midnight for crucial platelets or blood; juggling consulting physicians; consoling Barbara, the family and all her friends; seeing the regular office patients with cheerful mien; trying to teach the medical student; trying to maintain a normal, happy mood for my family; having dinner on the table at six o'clock; helping with homework not ignoring or denigrating the hurts borne by children growing up, even though a "more important" life or death matter hangs in the air—this multitudinous balancing act, for a moment, fell apart and all the balls went crashing to the floor in a heap.

He said, shocked and worried, "Mama! What's wrong?"

"Oh, nothing," I sobbed.

"Yeah, really—nothing," he said sarcastically, but gently,

The tears continued. I felt suspended in space, defeated. I stared at him. He looked at me searchingly, not saying a word for a long time. Then he asked softly, "Did your patient with the leukemia die?"

Of course, I thought, they all had heard me on the phone a hundred times, answering calls from the nurses at the hospital, or conferring with consultants—they all knew she existed, even my eight and ten-year-old daughters knew. I closed my eyes and nodded. He came up to me and put his arms around my neck and gave me a really tender squeeze and kissed my tear-flooded face.

"You really tried hard, Mama, I know you did. It's not your fault. It's no one's fault."

"I know," I said. "It's just that it's so unfair—if you had known her—just don't grow up thinking it's a fair world and maybe it won't hurt so much."

That was a lie. I had known from my earliest memories, from those concentration camp movies they showed during and just after the war, that it wasn't a fair world. And still it hurt—maybe even more, for it seemed that surely a quota must be reached sometime.

I hugged my small son desperately, a little ashamed of showing such weakness in front of him, and my tears stopped.

"You've helped me a lot," I said. "Thank you, angel—now, what can I make you for breakfast? You'll never catch the bus if we don't hurry. Is your bed made, your room picked up? Did you brush your teeth? Did you feed the dog? Please put out the garbage while I make your egg."

The phone rang while I was cooking, This was quite usual, and my long, coiled phone cord allowed me to cook in peace, while making medical decisions, Only rarely did I get the dose of a drug mixed up with the ingredients in a recipe. This time it was not the hospital but service telling me to call Barbara. I returned her call right away.

"Oh, Doctor," she said, her voice flattened with grief, but expressive, "I just had to call you to tell you how wonderful you've been through it all. I've so appreciated all the extra time you've spent, the way you cared so much about Molly. I know she appreciated it, too, We both knew how hard it's been for you." Again I was amazed; as I had been when Molly, having just heard she had leukemia, was feeling bad for me, that I was the one who had to tell her!

I said, with great difficulty keeping my voice steady, "Barbara, you were such a comfort to her, even though she was so strong, so serene. Molly was like a rock of strength—and all the nurses loved her. She knew how lucky she was to have a friend like you, and I've really appreciated your helping me in caring for her. I only wish things could have turned out differently—if only the drugs had worked."

Barbara's voice strengthened but cracked a little as she said, "Doctor, you know I've been thinking all along and even more so now—she might have had a remission, yes, but she would have been so weak after all she went through, and by the time she got her strength back she'd have a relapse, and we'd repeat it all again. All the suffering. Maybe it's for the best this way."

"Well, you do have a point," I conceded. "Maybe so."

I didn't really agree because I thought of the beautiful remissions I had seen during which the patients returned to normal life. But it comforted her to think so and who knew? Perhaps she was right.

"Please let me know if there's anything I can do for you, Barbara," I said. "I know it's going to be hard for you in the weeks ahead—getting used to the idea that she's really gone. Please do call me if you'd like, if you think I can help."

I was really worried about depression, for Molly was Barbara's significant "family," and now Barbara would be alone.

"Thank you Doctor. I promise I will. Bye!"

"Bye, Barbara."

The eggs and toast were ready. I had made four of each for all the children and my husband. I got dressed while they ate. I sketched in the events for my husband between his exit from the shower and his shave, on his way to the eggs, minus the emotional overtones since there was no time for such things,

We all left the house together, at 7:50 AM, on the day after Molly Lloyd died.

CHAPTER EIGHTEEN

Terror in the Office

It was an ordinary day in my family medicine practice, many years ago. A variety of patients, many long-standing and from various generations of whole families, filled the waiting room. Back then, I had four very efficient and nice women working for me, each with various duties. We had three examining rooms and a small lab. (Since, I've cut back but haven't left medicine yet!)

All of a sudden, looking panicky and terrified, my office manager burst into my private office where I was counseling a patient after her exam.

She said RL (not his real initials) was in the waiting room, waving around a knapsack full of guns, and threatening everyone!

She told me he wanted to see me immediately—and that he wanted *me* to take his guns away from him!

He had been a particularly difficult patient, but we had thought we were making progress with him.

He had an artificial leg (everyone thought he had been in Vietnam), but it had come from his intentionally running in front of a truck, trying to end his life. This was way before he became our patient.

He was found, by psychiatric consultation, to be psychotic (a condition of profound disordered thinking and/or feeling) but, when he was taking the right psychiatric medicines, he had many good and normal aspects of his nature. He didn't like the psychiatrist, and preferred to have me order his medicines.

Uh oh! He must be off his meds, I immediately figured. He had been taking pills, which he and I knew were helping to correct his faulty thinking, but was always forgetting to take them—so we arranged for him to have a shot weekly instead which was, at the time, an acceptable treatment. He had refused to see a psychiatrist regularly, preferring our welcoming office and more personal care, where we also accomplished his general medical care as well, as with any well-run family medicine practice.

I told my office manager to usher him into my office, while excusing the current patient who sat there, telling her that I would be with her just as soon as we were finished.

Meanwhile, I began trembling, trying to think fast with a perplexing mix of questions in mind as to how best to handle such an unexpected crisis.

I knew that he trusted me—that was why he had come. I knew that I shouldn't antagonize him at all, but I didn't know specifically what would set him off, or what would calm him down.

He was obviously relieved that the office manager would immediately take him to see me. I put on my best, relaxed greeting and told him we were happy to see him, since he needed a checkup anyway, which we could do today, since he had come. He did respond to being welcomed. He clutched his full canvas knapsack tightly.

I asked him right away if he had perhaps forgotten to go to the ER, where we had arranged the weekly anti-psychotic medicine shot.

"Yes," he said. "But I didn't forget. I just want to stop that medicine."

I asked what I could do to help him.

"Take these guns away from me. I'm afraid I might use them," he replied, and took one out and brandished it in front of me.

I sat still in my seat, behind my desk. *Is this the way it ends?* I wondered. I had read about doctors being shot by irate patients and I had no idea what would come next.

I tried my best not even to blink.

"RL," I said. "You know we've always wanted the best for you. We've taken good care of you."

"Yes, you have—that's why I'm here," he said. "I knew you'd fix it."

"Where did you get these guns?" I asked. "And how many are there? And why do you want me to take them away from you?"

He told me there were three pistols of various sizes, and a rifle. It was easy to get guns, he explained.

"Are you going to call the police?" he asked.

"I'm going to do whatever is best for you," I said. "You are my patient—for a long time now—and we want to help you. What do you think?"

"Take these away from me," he said. "I'm scared I might use them."

"Would you be willing to go straight from here to the ER where they have been giving you your medicine routinely from my order?" I asked him. "We will call ahead to be sure they will take you right away. You know you will feel more normal with it."

"Yes," he replied. "But it has some side effects that I don't like."

"We'll deal with that a little later, and maybe change to another just as good, okay?" I asked.

He stood up. I was still terrified. He reached down, replaced the pistol he had been holding in his hand inside the bag, picked up the long, canvas knapsack with the rifle and three pistols it, came around the desk as I stood up. He handed me the knapsack. It was so heavy, it took both hands to hold.

"You're doing the right thing, you know," I said, looking him in the eye.

"You're not going to call the police?" he asked again.

"I have no reason to. You're going along with the best plan to keep you and everyone else safe, and I am very happy with that. I want you to keep all your appointments, with me and with the psychiatrist. We really care about you and your treatment for your illness."

"I know," he said. "And that's why I came here. I feel better now."

I walked him out of the office, calmly, past all the staff and the other patients, half of whom had left in terror, not knowing what might happen next.

After an hour, I called the ER to verify that he had gone to get his shot. They said yes.

CHAPTER NINETEEN

Sudden, Somber Surprise

There is an art theater that plays foreign and unusual films on the university campus—the CD Theater. Every time I go to the CD with friends, instead of relaxing and enjoying the film, I relive the dark days that led to the theater's dedication and re-naming. Then, for him, CD, I do pay attention to the film; it is what he would have wanted.

For me, that dark time began just after I got home at the end of one usual day—examining and treating the customary array of patients. It was remarkable only in that the well thought they were especially sick, and the certifiably ill thought they were doing just fine.

The kitchen phone rang just as I had started dinner preparations. It was Lucy, and in the background, adding to all her comments, her husband Jack. They were begging me to do something, anything! They were worried about their good friend CD, who was a long-time patient of mine and a prominent film critic for the local newspaper. He should have arrived on a plane from New York, they told me, and they also said he was extremely ill, with a cough and fever, and his diabetes seemed out of control. They had exhorted him to seek medical care before leaving, and he said that his fiancé had told him the same thing. But he felt he would get better and opted to come home to Miami. He knew his doctor, he had a good support in the community, and he had work to do.

But Lucy said, they hadn't heard from him. His plane had landed hours ago, and they had been calling him, receiving no answer. They had been to his house, but couldn't tell if he was home, since the car was there, but they knew he had taken a cab to the airport and presumably one back home. He was not answering any doorbell, or responding to pounding on windows, whose curtains were drawn.

I told them to go back to CD's house in Coral Gables and stay there to await the police, whom I would call as soon as I hung up. But as I put down the phone, it rang again in my hand; it was my service with a call from the fiancée in New York. I debated for one second only, and then decided to call the police first.

I explained the situation and apologized in case it turned out to be a false alarm with an easy explanation, but I made it very clear that based on the facts, and my medical knowledge of CD, that he was likely in big trouble. I asked them to break into the house if necessary and said that his friends would be there waiting for them. The police sergeant hesitated, not knowing who I was, but I was aggressive, though polite in my depiction of the probable true urgency—if not emergency—of the situation. I said they could argue with me later, but please go now, since there was no time to spare, and if it was evident that CD needed immediate care, to take him to the nearest hospital in Coral Gables, which happened to be near his house and also to mine.

Then I called his fiancée. Actually, I felt I already knew her. CD had shown me her picture more than once, and—writer that he was—had waxed fairly poetic about how finally, at his age of forty-five, he had found someone not only that he was crazy about, but that he also wanted to marry. And she had found him. They were ecstatically happy and looking forward to a bright life ahead.

I explained to her that the delay in my calling back was because I was calling the police to assess the situation, and to break into the house if necessary. She was upset and crying, but I had to get a pertinent history from her, since she had been with him most recently. I told her that I could easily be wrong about him being in trouble, but just in case he was, he might need some attention. I wanted to prepare her for the worst while hoping for the best.

She portrayed a picture of him coughing, raising thick, yellow sputum, being short of breath, noting his sugars out of control, giving himself extra insulin, but worried about giving too much because his eating pattern was so irregular with the work he was doing. She had had grave misgivings about his getting on that plane, and she had told him that.

CD had come to me some ten years earlier, a vigorous, boyish, athletic and trim intellectual, who was also a regular guy. His was a rising star as the lead film critic for the prominent newspaper of the area. Everyone trusted his columns, which were witty, clever and right on the mark. I had diagnosed type 1 diabetes a few years back, but he was almost never sick. He was a maverick man-about-town, and enjoying every minute. But he had not found the soul mate he was looking for—until now. This was why on every visit he had to describe to me in his ebullient way how wonderful she was and how different and happy his life had become was, and how much he looked forward to their future together.

His two friends, Lucy and Jack, who had called me, were also sometime patients of mine; I knew them, but not as well as I knew CD. They were part of the theater-film-arts scene of the city, and were dependable buddies of CD. I knew that he would approve of involving them in his care. At the time, the new HIPAA laws concerning patient privacy were not in existence, and my sharing any of his details with them could today be construed as violating his privacy, But then, I decided that the emergency of the situation was enough to justify it. But what if there were no emergency? What if there was a simple explanation? Or even a complicated explanation? Possibly one that he wouldn't have wanted known to anyone?

I asked the officers to beep me as soon as they had any information, and that I would meet them at the hospital if needed. I refrained from going over to the house myself, realizing that if the police found him in distress or unconscious, or even dead, I would need to be at the hospital where he would be taken, which was closer to my house than his

Soon, I got a thinly-veiled, falsely calm call from the police trying to mask their urgency with their professionalism. They had broken into the house and found CD, wandering and stumbling around, confused and disoriented, very short of breath, barely able to give his name, and thoroughly incapable of calling for help. So, they had called rescue, which would arrive any minute.

I immediately called back his fiancée and told her that CD was very sick, but that we couldn't yet know how sick, and that she should catch the next plane down.

I got into my car, reviewing in my mind the treatment of diabetic ketoacidosis (something family doctors don't see every day) along with sepsis, likely from pneumonia, since these were my long-distance diagnoses before he was found, and I worried that my worst fears were coming true. I also got on the phone with my favorite endocrinologist, and asked her to meet me at the ER, sketching out the history, apologizing that I wouldn't ask her ordinarily but that this was a patient of utmost importance at a crucial time.

As I rushed into the ER and went up to CD, he saw me, recognized me, and said my name. He smiled weakly and said, "You're gonna pull me out of this, right, Doc?" I nodded, just as weakly, mustering an encouraging smile, barely believing that I would, or that anyone could pull him out of it, but not allowing myself to believe that we couldn't. He was indeed in florid ketoacidosis, but worse, he had overwhelming sepsis (widespread infection) from pneumonia, with total white-out of his entire right lung.

Superimposed on his gaunt, vacant face I could still see the vibrant, boyish, confident personage I had first met years ago, and had last seen only weeks before. I worked as though in a dream, hyper acutely, totally obsessed with doing everything right and not missing anything, but not really believing this was happening. Not to him. Not now—just when his happiness and his future were secured.

The word spread fast; Lucy and Jack had, of course, called all their friends and his bosses at the newspaper. The editors were swift in showing their concern, not just for him, but about whether he was getting the "best possible care." In consultation, we called a special physician not on staff at the hospital, giving him one-case privileges, because he was the chief at the big county hospital ER, reassuring the journalists that he was "the best." But I, as the generalist and his long-time personal physician, needed to make the difficult decisions, deciding which specialists to call in and pulling it all together. My role was inevitable, knowing CD well, knowing his friends, and now his fiancée. And with that central tenet—that I had to be the one to bear that honor and that responsibility—I became completely enmeshed in the case, unable to do almost anything else, until it defined itself, one way or another.

By then it was clear that CD was in full-blown adult respiratory distress syndrome, and I knew we might lose him. I was not comfortable with his being cared for at that hospital, although it was appropriately the closest for the emergency and in general was good. But it was not known for its Intensive Care as much as some other hospitals not far away. All the doctors on the case got together and debated whether to move CD or not.

Finally, we all came to agree that although moving him in an ambulance with a twenty-minute ride was a big risk (he could die on the way, and we could be faulted for ever having attempted to move him) nevertheless, once there, his care would involve much better round-the-clock (or twenty-four-hour) surveillance by special intensivists as well as more skilled nursing care.

He survived the move which was done with all equipment to keep everything going. In the new hospital he was placed with the most advanced team that could be mustered, and all the right treatments were given. Some worked; his sugar did normalize, but his blood pressure continued to drop, he could not be well-oxygenated, the sepsis was overwhelming, and finally, nothing helped.

By then, his fiancée, E, had arrived from New York. She was able to see him, still alive but unable to communicate. He was essentially comatose. I described his case in detail to her, what had probably happened before we rescued him, what had happened since, and what to expect. I explained the meaning of all things medical, and why he was in such dire straits. I hoped to deflect the inherent emotionalism into a clinical reality. I kept telling her that I had seen worse cases pull through, and whenever there were hopeful signs she would be kept informed. I explained that at least he was not suffering, he was not in pain. She was devastated, but I knew I had to prepare her for the possibility that such possible hopeful signs did not mean he would make it. Everyone became tired and then exhausted, keeping vigil night and day.

Despite all efforts we failed. I failed. CD died. The cause was septic shock, pneumonia, diabetic ketoacidosis, and adult respiratory distress syndrome. I had kept in such close touch with everyone that despite the overwhelming devastation and melancholy endured by all of us when the end finally came, his fiancée, and his friends thanked me profusely for all I had done for him, trying to make me feel better by telling me they knew we had all tried our best.

I was sent kind notes from E and her friends. I went to the funeral, where notables in journalism, politics, arts and theater gathered to mourn and eulogize him. He had been much loved and respected. Very shortly thereafter, they named the theater at the university for him.

For the next few weeks, I moved as in a daze. I had lost many patients in my medical lifetime, including a year in the early 1960s when in a cancer ward every patient was either dying or would soon die. I could usually do my grieving and get through it, even with patients with whom I had bonded and knew well. Somehow, this one was different.

I knew we had done everything. Really. I marveled that I had made the right moves as soon as I heard about it, calling the police, transferring him to a better facility, calling in whoever it took to be sure everyone's input was being respected, bonding with his fiancée and giving her support. I did a mental autopsy on the case from start to finish, over and over again, ruminating, rehashing. But my grief and yes—my doubt—did not let me alone.

After about three months, I realized that I was the one that needed support. My husband tried to reassure me, but I knew he couldn't know what it's like being in the middle of something like this case. Then a simple light bulb flashed in my head. I called up a good friend of mine, another family doctor. I told her I'd like to have lunch with her and needed to talk to her about something. Would she mind?

We met at a small café and had a sandwich. I proceeded to tell her the details of what had happened, how it all happened, and how strange and unrelentingly distraught I felt. I told her I was aware that something about this was different, that I couldn't let go. And I needed to let go. I needed some kind of insight into why I couldn't. As I talked I began to catch a glimmering, just a fragment of an idea that seemed as though it could be a key. It was elusive, as though it were a feather wafting in the air that I couldn't grab.

My friend was a very good listener. She then told me what I already knew to be fact. That my role had been important, that we had all the right consultations, that everything went as it should have, that no stone had been left unturned, that my relations with everyone were impeccable, that everyone was understanding and even grateful. I think I told her that I knew all this with my mind, but I didn't feel it with my heart. And worse, I didn't know why I couldn't feel it. But I was happy to be recounting everything, telling it all to someone who was just there to give me support.

I began to catch hold of the elusive thought, the insight. It was this: my confidence had been shaken, almost broken. The experience was so dreadful that I doubted my ability and my own validity. I knew this wasn't about me, it was about him, and now he was gone. So it became about me. But if he were still here, even he would say that we all did what we should have done and could have done.

I began to tell myself that the biggest tribute to him would be if his case could give me more confidence, not less. That is what he would have wanted. He would want me to let go of my obsessive grief. He would want that my ability and validity be measured not by whether he lived or died, but by how we had cared for him—not by winning but by how we had played the game.

CHAPTER TWENTY

A Mango for Meemo

It is summer, and mango season. She sits staring as I walk in with the mangos. The look is as blank as flat concrete. I steel myself for the sheering force of the shell my mother has become. She may take my hand and say my name. Or she may say, "Who is this? This place isn't for you. Go home." With all the Alzheimer's patients I have had in my family practice, you would think I would be prepared for this turmoil.

Having her at our home seemed the right thing to do after her adoring new husband of three years could not care for her. She had called me daily at the office saying he was trying to kill her. I had to baby-proof the house as though a toddler lived there. She was up all night wandering around. Medications for sleep made her stagger, those for agitation made her nauseated.

She often thought I was trying to harm her. Once she came at me and grabbed my face with her fingernails, twisting my cheek like a cat fight among girls. I screamed for my husband, unwilling to fight my tiny mother. A minute later she hugged me and told me how much she loved me—what blessed forgetfulness. This was my sweet mother who had kissed my forehead when I was a child and who told and retold the story of how I was burning up with fever as I was bundled off to the hospital, aged four, temperature 106 degrees Fahrenheit. I had typhoid fever when there was no treatment for it. Several children in that mini-epidemic on Miami Beach had died. And she kept asking my father, "What if she dies? What if she dies?" And every time she told the story, tears would softly stream from her eyes, but she held them back so they never fell onto her cheeks.

These days my mother often looks at me with expressions identical to those of when she was normal. I look into her eyes and can no longer fathom the blankness I know is there. It is the mirror of the piercing stare of a newborn who seems to know what you are thinking. I am learning what the families of my patients come to know while they are suffering: They are doing their grief work in advance.

I bring her mangos, her favorite fruit—mine, too.

"Do you know what I brought you, Meemo?" I ask (she was renamed 'Meemo' long ago by a grandchild).

"Why do you ask such a stupid question?" she asks. "I don't know, and I don't care." She does not recognize the mangos.

"Remember how Daddy used to plant fish heads under the mango tree to fertilize it?" I ask. This is one of our favorite family secrets. She pushes the mangos away. I go to the kitchen of the house where she lives and peel a mango, fighting the same tears she always fought.

This is not about you, I admonish myself; *this is about her.*

I bring the plate of mangos with a fork. She will not touch them. I force a jolly smile and pierce a piece of mango, bringing it to her lips, as she must have done for me as an infant. She licks it, then opens her mouth like a little bird.

She knows the mango!

She takes the fork, a smile spreading over her face. She gobbles down the plate of mangos, grinning as the juice runs down her chin.

My mother was a no-nonsense, practical lady, but she was sentimental. She was cute and quick and had written a book of poetry that she refused to call by that name. She called it verse and said she was a versifier, not a poet. Some verses were one-liners: "Life is a dress rehearsal for which there will never be an opening night." She could not have known how slowly and painfully the curtain would descend and that the theater would be empty before the stage lights would finally go out.

Until then, I will bring her mangos or whatever else is in season.

Activism and Writing

CHAPTER TWENTY-ONE

The Real Drama

It is a perpetual, exhausting question: how can we motivate patients to do what they need to do soon enough not to end up in a situation requiring preventable, heroic attempts to save them? Often there are powerful forces, either within families or out in society, pulling in the direction of self-destruction, towards either excessive thinness or fatness: food tastes good, advertising (either for food or for figure) is persuasive, eating confers conviviality, warmth and social acceptance. Eating is a source of love and pleasure. So are living and breathing.

The concept of delayed gratification (the difference between an adult and a child) is clear to most. People work hard, saving for a secure future. Where eating is concerned, they may revert to childish ways: I want what I want, when I want it. The discipline and thought to the future evaporates.

Popular images thrust upon people by the advertising age nudge the subconscious: "things go better with Coke," "aren't you hungry?" "where's the beef?," "finger-lickin' good," "fine dining for connoisseurs," or—in the case of anorexia— "you can't be too rich or too thin." Where are the advertising images connecting habits with health? Perhaps in a few athletic shoe ads: just do it. Mostly these messages are absent, unless there's a product to sell.

Those in charge of the national budget for "health care" do not have the imagination to devote a tiny percentage of what is now granted to research, sick care and cure, for other strategies. Enough is already known about behavior, disease processes, motivation and advertising to put some of that knowledge to work. Mass media appeal regularly creates fads overnight.

An ongoing multimedia strategic campaign for healthy behavior would help as much as medical care, and would cost less.

To our credit, there *is* more health awareness in this country than others. This may be partly because of the very personal medical system prevailing here until now. But the inroads of canned care, though claiming to be interested in "health maintenance," discourages doctors from seeing patients often enough to know what's happening with them, since it gives incentives *not* to see patients.

The aim is "reducing costs," read maximizing profits, of the companies, or minimizing costs to government. If a clinic is government-run, only screening tests which can be justified by large "controlled" studies showing dollar-yield per patient are deemed advisable. The study has not and likely could not be done to reveal the difference in the health and timely treatment of persons whose doctors know them well, provide continuity through long years, and care about them and their families.

THE DOCTOR ASKED JOE, his impatient patient, to sit down and not to worry about the others waiting, that this extra time was worth it—to both of them. The doctor told Joe about the patient in the ICU, and described the scene in the ER the night before. He told him that today Joe's bronchitis brought him in—but he won't die of it. He explained that what he might die of might not bring him in until he's too sick to do much about it. He asked Joe to come back for a complete physical and fasting blood profile, at which time other non-cardiac early detection/prevention methods could also be advised.

The doctor said that the Joe's thinking, feeling and behaving about *food* and *eating* may be in his own power, right now. Once Joe makes a decision that it's worth it to change his outlook, many methods of modifying behavior can work. The doctor could help him there. But the *decision* is Joe's.

The doctor tried to get him to see some of the subtle forces causing him to do what *isn't* best for him, and that he doesn't have to be acted upon by those forces, but can *decide* to be healthy. He tried to get Joe to see that the chest-thumping, hair-raising, heroic scene of last night's adventure may be the stuff of which TV movies are made. Yet taking a little extra time even in the middle of a busy day like today—repetitious and boring as it was for the doctor, tedious and preachy for the patient—this was where the plot could be changed and the storybook ending achieved. This was the real drama.

Note: Most articles on eating disorders pertain to anorexia, rather than obesity or hyperlipidemia, which, though there are significant genetic components, are also eating disorders in most cases. The points made here—*that prevention is as important as treatment*—pertain to nearly every disease entity. Though treatment gets more attention, better methods of early detection and prevention are where the real drama lies.

The Demise of the Independent Doctor: A Self-Fulfilling Prophecy?

ABSTRACT: Most physicians wish to preserve their freedom and autonomy not only for themselves but in order to deliver the best medical care. Some physicians together with businesspeople/bureaucrats are engaged in subtle attempts to eliminate the relatively independent and autonomous practice of medicine. Yet when physicians join together to preserve their individual freedom, they could be accused of antitrust activities. A whole profession may be losing its nobility and mobility on the altar of the dollar. "Managed" health care in whatever form (government or corporate) can exist beside autonomous and independent medical care without overwhelming the system, but only if physicians beware the self-fulfilling prophecy that independent medicine is dead, by actively and innovatively rejecting the false and misleading "hype" which surrounds them. Medical organizations nationwide, instead of following trends, should be taking the lead to preserve freedom for doctors and patients.

Among the "junk" mail were two slick brochures, the design imaginative, paper unique, printing impressive. One touted the organizer-MD's expertise at teaching us to work within HMOS, IPAS, PPOS. The other proposed to tell us what medicine will be like in the year 2000. One slogan was, "Don't miss this opportunity to learn about the future of medicine," the other, "Changing relationships between hospitals and physicians."

We, ourselves, become led and misled by the hype.

Some of our own physicians-turned-businessmen/bureaucrats plus genuine businesspeople/bureaucrats are engaged in subtle attempts to band together to eliminate the relatively-independent and autonomous practice of medicine; yet when we join together (though apart) to preserve our individual freedom, we could be accused of antitrust activities!

Many of us form a silent majority who know that it is not only our self-interest as physicians which is at stake but the dismantling of the fine medical system we have known.

Freedom and Autonomy: uses and abuses ✦ Most of us who practice medicine in the real world wish to preserve the freedom and autonomy of individual physicians. We have the old-fashioned belief that this is genuinely the best way to give medical care to people.

Multiple problems involve not just physical illnesses but other factors in peoples' lives; their physician becomes their true advocate, who can move freely within whatever systems are involved with getting what they need and making them well.

Most physicians used to feel this way. Now many say freedom is dead (a self-fulfilling prophecy?).

Sadly, a few, but very few, physicians abuse their freedom and also abuse the third-party payer systems, especially Medicare, which physicians opposed originally knowing it would lead to cost overruns. These physicians over-charge and over-utilize, wishing to be free so that "no one will look over their shoulder." So it happens that politics makes strange bedfellows: those who welcome scrutiny may ally with those who have something to hide.

Costs and causes ✦ Data show that costs of our entire "medical system" are due mostly to hospitals and other medical business charges including health insurance and professional liability insurance. Physicians' over-utilization and over-charging must be a fraction of the problem since only 19% to 21% of the entire medical costs "pie" represents all physician charges. A hue and cry from the public goes out that the entire system is now unaffordable. Therefore we must ensnare all doctors to work within some sort of controlled and "managed" health care scheme. This throws the baby (maintenance of freedom and autonomy for physicians for the benefit of patients) out with the bath water (the morass of cost overruns and over-utilizations, which weren't attributable to most doctors in the first place).

And if over-supply of physicians is a problem, and some of us are struggling, how can more middlemen (administrators) splitting the medical dollar be of help?

There are segments of the population who, for whatever reason, are willing to compromise their care. They and their employees wish to pay less. They can get fairly adequate medical care through various organizational schemes.

This is the HMO concept and we need not oppose this as one of the alternatives in medicine.

Having an HMO as an alternative is far different from having the concept become the only, albeit less desirable, means of delivery of medical care.

Conflicts, capture and Control ♦ The doctors who work in the HMO, IPA, and even PPO framework can never be true patient advocates because they do not have true freedom themselves. There are conflicts of interest constantly hamstringing them right down to the loss of their very jobs and/or their patient base. Patients need to know this.

Follow the logic of an HMO organizer. 1. Independent doctors really are better for free people. 2. When doctors are independent some may charge too much. 3. People cannot afford to pay too much. 4. Although most overpricing has not been due to physicians in the first place, let's entice doctors by offering to "help" them. 5. We will take their patients. 6. We will give the patients back to the doctors through well paid middlemen (some of whom are doctors, themselves). They will have control of every aspect of medical care and a share of every dollar spent.

The people will say they are paying less; they won't know they are getting less. The doctors will say they are getting "fee for service." But once the patient population has been "captured" and enrolled in a large organization which sets a fee schedule and doles out money and medical care according to its own decisions, the doctor who for a while was satisfied will be completely within the "managed" health care sphere. The doctor (and the patient) will be unable to move in either direction. They will have lost their power, control and cash flow.

Same lorry—different driver ◆ This is the case with socialized medical schemes as well as with corporate medical schemes and it does not matter who controls it; doctors, businessmen or bureaucrats. The individual physician and patient will still be in a "managed" health care scheme In the words of an African song: Same lorry (truck)—different driver.

Territorial imperative ◆ Abraham Lincoln, in 1859, was running for president.

The debate was: should slavery, though it was entrenched in the south, be allowed to spread into the Federal Territories?

This is what Abraham Lincoln had to say.… "wrong as we think slavery is, we can yet afford to let it alone where it is because that much is due to the necessity arising from its actual presence in the nation; but can we, while our votes will prevent it, allow it to spread into the National Territories, and to overrun us here in these free states? If our sense of duty forbids this, then let us stand by our duty fearlessly and effectively."

He reasoned: "…their thinking it right and our thinking it wrong, is the precise fact upon which depends the whole controversy. Thinking it right, as they do, they are not to blame for desiring its full recognition, as being right; but thinking it wrong, as we do, can we yield to them? Can we cast our votes to their view, and against our own?" He finished, "Let us have faith that right makes might and in that faith let us, to the end, dare to do our duty as we understand it."

Just as we should acknowledge that HMOS, IPAS and other schemes for managed health care may have the their place and their advocates, we should fight for not letting them spread out of the territory which they now occupy into the larger territory of independent medicine, itself, and certainly not by our own hand through our own medical organizations.

"Our duty as we understand it" ◆ We need to put out a call to organized and unorganized medicine all over this country, even though we know that certain county and state medical organizations have legitimized the concept by forming their own ipas, hmos and ppos. We need to put out a call to doctors who have not joined with organized medicine, partly because they have felt that organized medicine has done and can do nothing for them. Perhaps if they realize the firm stand that we will take for the independent doctor they will close ranks with us. This is not to say that doctors who work within the hmos and ipas should be disenfranchised. Organized medicine should stand for individual physicians wherever they are, within whatever system they practice. But the concept that hmos and ipas exist should not imply that they will sweep this country and it won't, unless we allow it to happen. There is still time left.

By limiting individual autonomy we will become enslaved and ensnared in managed health care which ultimately will not benefit our individual and free patients.

Finding solutions ◆ Well, you say, what are the alternatives? There are many; we need only to find them. That is where we should be putting our efforts. Many organizations are cropping up around the country with the sole aim of preserving independent medical practice.

The most important corollary will be that we—if we choose to remain independent doctors—will have to act responsibly and never allow ourselves to succumb to the temptation of over-utilization and excessive pricing in the field of medicine. Physicians in technical specialities and for-profit ventures in which it is possible to accumulate great wealth by "practicing medicine" should rethink their positions very carefully. A whole profession may be losing its nobility and mobility on the altar of the dollar.

Plans in perspective ◆ For a young doctor coming out of training, an hmo, like military service, is an opportunity to work, earn money and get his/her feet wet in medicine. He/she will soon realize, as I did, working in various "jobs" in medicine, (city health departments, maternal and child health clinics, college health services and other forms of managed health care) that in no case is he/she allowed to be a true advocate of his/her patients.

He will yearn for the autonomy that he knows he requires in order to do right by his patients.

He will then go into practice, perhaps on a shoe string. He will spend a few years not making much money because his practice is young, and then he will make a reasonable living and support his family not with great wealth but with adequacy.

Some people may elect to stay in managed health care schemes. This is fine but there should be the other option of being an independent doctor among free people.

The media and the message ◆ We should be looking for innovative means of delivering this and similar messages to our own doctors and to the public. We should be involved in lowering total medical costs for patients. We should not be involved in plans for setting up subgroups within our medical organizations which stand to gain economically from investing in IPAS and HMOS and whose administrators will, of course, be paid for their efforts and will form another wedge between the doctor and the patient.

"Doctor-controlled and doctor-owned" has very little meaning in this context. No matter who controls it, you the physician will not have a voice and the steamroller will roll over you (and your patients). I believe that there are a lot of us out there—perhaps a silent majority—who agree.

Speak up and speak out ◆ Why must we acquiesce so easily? Why must we believe the advertisements that we hear on TV and radio when we know differently? In this age of media madness, why must we be part of a self-fulfilling prophecy? Why must we join every plan for fear of being left out, instead of remaining resolutely free of such encumbrances?

Perhaps we simply have not managed our own media approach to ourselves properly. Perhaps we don't have the collective confidence and will.

I think we do. Think it over. Are you part of that silent majority? If so, speak up and speak out—now before it's too late.

I think we should beware of self-fulfilling prophecies. We may be down but we're not out. But if we lie down and let the HMO, IPA and other "managed" schemes roll over us, we will get what we deserve because we haven't fought the fight and the face of medicine will be changed forever.

CHAPTER TWENTY-THREE

The March to Tallahassee

This is the story of a huge, successful gathering by doctors from all over Florida at the state capitol in 1986, also joined by businesses being buried by insurance and malpractice inequities, to repeal the onerous law made the year before and about to go into effect, mandating malpractice insurance as condition of medical licensure. We were inspired by doctors in New York and Illinois who marched to their state capitols and got results.

Repealing the law would allow competence and training to continue to be the criteria for a doctor to hang a shingle, not the ability to buy commercial insurance. There was also the element of placing a cap on non-economic damages in malpractice law suits.

Most unbelievably, the entire march was begun by the efforts of two doctors—one of them myself—not by our medical association, who declined (at first) to attempt to mobilize, opining that apathy and unwillingness to get involved among doctors would preclude any useful action.

This will include a preamble recounting invited public debates with the most prominent malpractice attorney after I wrote an op-ed piece published as lead article in the *Miami Herald* op-ed section, March 17, 1985, refuting the attorney's vitriolic claims of the prior weeks' op-ed piece about "bad" doctors, reacting to an admittedly disastrous medical error at our large county hospital

ONE DAY IN 1985 I was giving a talk at a medico-legal seminar when the malpractice insurance crisis in Florida was in full swing. The legislature had just passed a law to go into effect January 1987 that doctors must buy malpractice insurance as condition of licensure. By then I had become somewhat known in the medical and legal community as having either spoken against or written against a lot of what was happening regarding medical malpractice that was adverse for physicians—especially for me—since insurance had risen sky-high, and I was a mother with three children and limited office-hours, though full-time availability as an active family physician.

I knew that if that law passed, I would become a non-physician. There was no way I could afford the insurance at the time. I had thought being a physician depended on training and competence, not on ability to ante up money into a corrupt and unconscionable dysfunctional "system" of "malpractice insurance."

I had written a response to a headline article by J.B. Spence, the feared and leading malpractice attorney in Miami-Dade County. His article was in the Sunday *Miami Herald* opinion section. He titled it in big headlines: "The Bad Side of Medicine." To blast all doctors, he had taken advantage of a tragic, accidental injection of formaldehyde into a well-known patient's spinal canal instead of anesthesia. The year was 1985.

My piece was longer than just a letter to the editor, and I challenged them to publish it the following Sunday, since they saw fit to publish such a diatribe, most of it either false or twisted. They called me from the *Herald* editorial department, not only wanting to publish it, unedited, in the same headline spot in the *Herald*, but offering to pay me for it! I accepted and donated the payment to a journalism scholarship. I titled it: "The Good Side of Medicine."

I was then asked to debate, by the same editor, the great J.B. Spence, himself, which I did (reluctantly and fearfully) to a packed house at a local venue. That's another David/Goliath vignette, but all my doctor-friends said that I "won" the debate.

But back to the medico-legal seminar where I was speaking that day: when I got through, a doctor who had been in the audience came up to me and said, "Hello. I'm Simon," with a charming South African accent.

"You're just what we need to spread the word about how wrong this is and how we have to change it."

I said, "Hi, and thank you. But what do you mean?"

He told me he was an anesthesiologist at "my" hospital, South Miami Hospital, and I realized I knew him by reputation and on paper, but had not really met him, and also that he was the husband of a fellow family physician in our department who I knew from our FP meetings.

Simon said, "Most of the doctors don't even know this law was passed and will go into effect January, 1987, and they have no idea what the implication for their practices and their lives will be. And besides—it's just wrong."

I said, "As you can tell from my talk, I thoroughly agree. But what can we do?"

"We can march to Tallahassee," he said.

"Haven't you heard?" I asked. "Don't you know getting doctors to do anything together is like herding cats?"

"Yes, but we could do it," he said. "Together, we could do it—but you would be essential."

Dumbfounded I asked, "Why?"

"Because you speak very well," he said. "You're very convincing and credible, and I know you could do it—we could do it."

"It's our medical organizations that should be taking this up," I said. "That's what they're for. Talk to our President of the DCMA." (Dade County Medical Association) He said that they only fight battles they think they have a good chance of winning. And this wouldn't be one of them.

Truth to tell, I was instantly intrigued, and intuitively knew I had the bull-dogging intenseness and stick-to-it-iveness for it, but not the organizational or logistic skills. I wouldn't have known where or how to start. And I told him so.

I was already somewhat active in the DCMA; little did I know then I was destined to become the Editor of our County Medical Journal, *Miami Medicine*, for three years, from 1992-1995. Then, in 1985, I was on a mediation committee and some other committee. One night, when I was at a meeting at their building downtown, the president of the DCMA, who, from my viewpoint, was always condescending to women in medicine in those days, was hanging out in the kitchen, where snacks were provided. Simon was there and we decided to ask him if he would organize the type of thing we had in mind, if he would get the organization to vote on it and do it. He said herding cats won't work. They've tried it before—never worked, and that the Florida Medical Association felt the same way. We're stuck with the law, period. Forget it. So we hemmed and hawed, gave evidence as we saw it that it was dead wrong, and tried to convince him otherwise, but he was adamant. They would not put any of their "resources" to it.

So then we asked the cutting question.

"Would you, as President, permit us to do it?"

He thought for a minute—and so convinced that it would go nowhere—said, "Well—Sure, go ahead and try. I don't advise it. But don't expect a penny of support from here. I won't tell you not to, but we won't fund it in any way nor vote on it either."

So Simon and I were on our own. We were not prohibited—but we were not supported. We considered this a huge victory. We were elated. Intuitively we realized that had they taken it over, they might have dropped the burden, but knowing if we did ourselves, we'd carry the ball as far as it needed. We'd find creative ways to get to goal.

We set ourselves tasks: make a list of all hospitals in the whole county; call their staff offices; get permission for five to ten minutes only to speak to the entire staff at their next meeting re: "the malpractice crisis and the new law"; bring a simple form to sign doctors (and others) to commit to putting their warm bodies where their mouths were and, along with the rest of us, to get on a plane to Tallahassee when the legislature is in session; reason with them from their perspectives—and ours; agree that we'd all like to carry such insurance, but that to make it mandatory without alternatives would be to capture our noble profession and render our MD useless in many cases.

This was before PowerPoint was even invented, so I prepared an easel, with many large turn-able pages, on which—in BIG LETTERS—were listed the precepts, ideas and steps to take in order to convince our legislators than this was an ill-conceived law, and how they could make it fair and better.

Then we trekked out to do the job. In each venue we were surprised at how well we were received, and many doctors agreed immediately, happy someone was taking action. They signed up then and there.

After two or three weeks, we had almost enough commitments to fill an airplane, and we got Jeb Bush, who was head of the Republican Party then in Miami, and Richard Pettigrew who was head of the Democratic Party here, to endorse what we were doing. Jeb ultimately rode up on the plane with us.

When the fma (Florida Medical Association, who had simply considered the law a "done deal") found out that we were actually doing this, the President and all the officers and staff jumped on board, spread the idea to all counties in Florida, and decided a statewide assembly in Tallahassee would be even more effective. They agreed to add businesses and executives who were struggling under equally onerous laws and obstructions that were benefitting lawyers and insurance companies, but not professionals and businesses, or even patients.

Then we went!

The doctors honored their commitments, paid their own way, and we flew to Tallahassee on a chartered plane—and so did most of the counties in Florida. Simon and I were very happy.

We marched up the hill to the capitol building. I marched with a roofer who was there because his business was chafing under legal and insurance requirements. We clogged the halls and offices of the building, speaking politely but convincingly to legislators and their staffs—urging them to repeal the mandatory law to buy insurance, while allowing physicians to "go bare" with certain assurances for patient safety.

The law was repealed. A reasonable law took its place, leaving a choice to "go bare" if need be.

CHAPTER TWENTY-FOUR

Poison Lampposts:
How to Lose the Battle and Win the War

*The recent tobacco-war triumphs did not occur in a
vacuum; they were and continue to be incremental, with
many small victories behind them. This was one.*

The lampposts were poisoned; there was no doubt.

As surely as if it were a terrorist target, they were the straight aim of premeditated murder, and the enslavement of the brave people of our town. They appeared overnight as though by stealth. The worst of it was that they had been there the year before. She thought her letter to the editor had squelched them for all time. *How naïve that was.* As though just pointing out the danger would be enough. As though elected city, county and state officials would have taken notice, just because the newspaper editor did.

All things pondered, they were the ones responsible, those officials. They gave the permits—they allowed it to happen. One couldn't blame nefarious forces and greedy commercial interests for being who and what they were; one could only blame those who failed to realize it and failed to take obvious action.

The poisoned lampposts were all the more dangerous because they were so attractive. The melding of artistic design with the most danger-ous substance known to cause more human death and destruction than any consumed chemical was sickening, yet strangely spell-binding.

The event connected with the lampposts, indeed advertised by them, was an exciting road race, and the lampposts were insidiously insinuating that the excitement and relative safety of the drivers and spectators could spill over into users of the product, and one could be proud and important while using it. The meanness of the subtleties and their implied and asserted meanings assaulted her senses, and her indignation grew incrementally as she passed each blurred post, driving swiftly down the highway, until her indignation turned to anger, then disbelief—to rage, then outrage. She could feel and taste the poison dripping from the lampposts. The poison was palpable.

That's when she swung into action. She realized she had to get them off those lampposts, one way or another. She had to make a huge splash or they would go on, year after year, after year. A brave protest, a letter to the paper, a mere calm pointing out of the danger wouldn't fill the bill. This had to be all-out war.

First, she called the city paper's publisher, whom she had met and interviewed for an article in her own local medical association magazine, which she had edited. Calling an editor was not her style; she always sent letters without prior contact or any attempt to influence, letting them stand on their own. This time was different; now results were needed, and time was important. The advertised race event had become another race. The lamppost poison had to be removed before the event they advertised, so that the perpetrators would be taught a lesson, and so that their expensive sponsorship would be in ruins. There was another dilemma here complicating the issue: the racetrack was a new addition to a smaller city within the larger county that was struggling with the recent upheaval following removal of an important air base, due to a devastating hurricane. She deeply respected that city's need to succeed, and the economic importance of the race, but she had a different race in mind: a race to the finish line of health and freedom from black death of the beloved citizens of her own town.

Driving down the highway, her thoughts and emotions swirled at her first glimpse of the poisoned lampposts. First was the new dilemma, the shock of being ignored. The realization that a just cause had been thwarted, the personal and professional necessity to favorably influence the health of the public and of her patients. Then came the visions, faces and remembrances of all the lung cancer deaths she had guided, and all she had prevented, the indignation borne of misplaced delusions of influence, the gauntlet thrown down for a challenge, the sweet pre-taste of victory, the glory of righteousness.

Luckily, it was neither fame nor fortune that motivated her, or she would have been sorely disappointed. As it turned out, others claimed the prize, chimed in on the chorus and shouted from the rooftops that if it hadn't been for their spotting the iniquitous enemy, and the initiation of opposition at their behest, there would not have been the victory. Their participation was crucial; that was accurate. Possibly without them, the goal would never have been reached. That they spread the word wonderfully, in the best possible way once it started, was undeniable. But she and they knew very well the truth of who gathered together the war chest of talent, who started the campaign, who followed it through, and whose victory it really was, and that was enough for her.

This is her account of what happened:

The time-line: (we suggest the use of a fictitious cigarette name in the final version of this article so as not to advertise further the poison about which we speak here):

March 1995: The Miami Grand Prix, a new road race sponsored by "Dover" Cigarettes puts up posters and banners all over the city of Miami and the county of Dade. There is a pack of cigarettes complete with the logo, name, colors and style of the actual pack thinly disguised as a race car, with the date and venue. It is repeated over and over again on almost all the large, tall lampposts—streetlights—of the city, including down u.s. 1, also known as Dixie Highway, in the south end of the county.

March 3, 1995: Letter to the Editor, the *Miami Herald*, headlined, "Don't use public assets to tout smoking."

> Dear Editor:
> As a physician who convinces people that they should quit tobacco use, who treats tobacco's devastating consequences, and who grieves with families over completely preventable premature deaths, I protest the abuse of city and county power by allowing Marlboro signs to dominate and pollute the landscape of our beautiful and healthy county. These signs are posted on our own lampposts all over Miami and county, and I, who

own them along with all residents, strongly object to "renting" those posts for this purpose.

This is not a First Amendment issue, but rather a public matter. Our own state is suing tobacco companies to recover billions in smoking-related costs.

The Miami Grand Prix notwithstanding, Marlboro's sponsorship should not include this type of flagrant abuse of public property. This sets a precedent: who next on our lampposts? The summit was the first, but it was a completely different concept. Take those posters down now! Don't wait for a lawsuit. Every day they do damage to impressionable new smokers and reinforce old ones.

Advertising works. Money talks. This campaign should not be yelling louder than the public's health, or with the complicity of county officials.

Very truly yours, PG, MD

The Grand Prix goes on as planned. The lampposts are thus decorated, long after the event. The damage is done, day by day. Those like-minded and I grit our teeth, confident that after it is over, it would not, could not happen again.

February 8, 1996: The signs—the same signs—go up again!

February 8, 1996: E-mail to *Miami Herald*: Copy of last year's letter. They edit it down but publish it urgently the next day, after the publisher receives my indignant call.

February 9, 1996: Letter to the Editor, the *Miami Herald*, headlined: No to Marlboro ("Dover") Banners:

Dear Editor:
As a physician who convinces people that they should quit using tobacco, treats tobacco's devastating consequences, and grieves with families over completely preventable premature deaths, I protest the abuse of city and county power by allowing Marlboro signs on lampposts to pollute our county's landscape This is not a first amendment issue; it's a public-health matter. Our own state is suing tobacco companies to recover billions in smoking-related Medicaid costs.

The Miami Grand Prix's sponsorship should not include this type of flagrant abuse of public property. Do the right thing: take down those Marlboro banners now. PG, MD

February 12, 1996: Letter to the County Manager, and all commissioners, with a copy faxed to Governor Lawton Chiles, all Florida legislators, the Mayor of City of Miami, the Mayor of County of Dade, etc., demanding that something be done within three days to answer the long list of specific questions designed to reveal who, in fact, was responsible, and by what authority, to grant such poisoning of our own lampposts.

February 13, 1996: Gary Nelson of Channel 4 contacts me, re: letter in paper (unaware of my faxes to County Manager, Governor, etc., asking who was responsible).

He interviews me on camera at my office, as part of a very effective story that runs at 6:00 PM (with a short version at 11:00 PM), exposing the irony of the state suing tobacco companies, and then letting them advertise on its own lampposts. (They find out that it is State right-of-way, not County). It seems the City of Homestead got a permit from the DOT (Department of Transportation, a so-called "courtesy" permit!!), and then contracted with someone to put them up. It also seems that the regulations of DOT specifically prohibit political or commercial messages on their rights of way.

Other TV channels come to the office to tape segments. Channel 4 runs another story stating that it was they who notified the Governor, ran the story, and made him aware of the problem!

February 14, 1996: Happy Valentine letter to County Manager.

> Dear Mr. Vidal:
> Happy Valentine's Day. This is a love-note to my beloved Dade County.
> Please see attached e-mail re: "Poison lampposts"
> Despite my error in assuming the county was responsible for posting the banners, nevertheless, this is occurring in our county. You, the mayor, and the commissioners are still responsible for what goes on here, and for staying on top of the state's responsibility to adhere to its own regulations.

My outrage is that it happened last year—was brought to everyone's attention—and for all I know, would have gone on year after year, had not one little person out here gotten very worked up about it.

I'm only writing to reinforce that it's not over yet. The banners are still up. Please consider it your and the county commission's job to work with the state to get them down urgently. Every minute is valuable advertising time which is paid for with the lives and health of our people. As a physician, I know this personally.

Thank your very much for your attention. I do *not* have the staff of facilities to copy all the commissioners again. I hope you will do so for me. Very truly yours,

PG, MD

February 15, 1996: Open letter to Governor Chiles and Officials of Dade County:

Gary Nelson of Channel 4 followed up on the saga of the poisoned banners, ending his story with a statement saying that the Governor said he would not take down the signs because it would be "unfair to the city of homestead and the grand prix." I am hoping the Governor did not mean that. Excuse me—but this is all about how unfair anyone and everyone who caused those signs to be up is to all the people. Whether or not the state is engaged in a suit against tobacco companies is irrelevant; it simply makes for irony. The fact is: the signs are advertising a commercial product, and a dangerous one at that, injuring the public's health, every minute they stay up.

Please don't talk about fairness in the same breath as you aid and abet a killing substance, on our tax-paid lampposts. Even if there were no regulation which the state itself violated, it would be against the health and well being of our community, and therefore ought not to be allowed by our officials without our permission. As I already said in another letter, if funds to take them down is the problem, I'm sure we can mobilize all the people in the county who *understand how poisonous tobacco is* to help take them down.

This is like saying, "we apprehended the wrong man, we made a colossal mistake, but we're going to jail him anyway because it would be unfair to the police who worked so hard to catch him." Please don't make lack of logic follow *your* colossal mistake.

Please take those banners down *now*. Every minute counts. Think what advertisers pay for critical minutes on tv. They know that it sells their product and brainwashes anyone who views it.

I appreciate everything Channel 4 has done to support this cause—and I certainly don't wish the City of Homestead any harm, since the city IS its people, and I am *defending* the health and lives of its people. I favor and support the Grand Prix.

But poisoned lampposts??? No thank you.

Remember, this is not new this year. The same letter that triggered this action was also in the paper last year at this time. Then there was not enough time to take down the banners. The outrage is that they are up again. Don't double the unfairness by refusing to take them down. *Now there is* enough time if you get started urgently.

If you do not, it means that money is talking much louder than the people's lives and health. Very truly yours, pg, md

To reiterate: Signs advertising the event are acceptable. Signs depicting and stating the name, logo and pictures of cigarettes are not acceptable. pg, md

February 16, 1996: More letters, back and forth, to the Mayor of Homestead, other officials, etc. Many letters and faxes to me from people (known and unknown to me) who are behind the effort, including a personal letter from Stanley Rosenblatt, the chief lawyer for the class action suits involving flight attendants and others in the State of Florida, encouraging our involvement.

February 18, 1996: Article in the *New York Times* Sunday paper, Nation Section, page 16, headlined, "In Florida, Do Banners Sell Racing, Or Tobacco?"

Dateline Miami, February 17: Quoting a spokeswoman for the Governor: "I seriously doubt you will see those banners next year."

The article ends: "After the race last year, Dr. Pepi Granat, a family doctor in South Miami, began a letter-writing campaign to prevent the banners from being used again. While Dr. Granat sees the race as a good event, she said she was upset by what she called the promotional effect. When the banners reappeared this year, she was one of the first to protest.

'These are poisoned lampposts,' she said. 'We should not be aiding and abetting a dangerous substance on our lampposts.'

February 19, 1996: Two letters in the Herald, one accusing me of hurting the economic well being of the city of Homestead, sent by the organizer of the Grand Prix.

February 19, 1996: Fax from me to Governor Chiles, with copies to the Commissioners, the *Miami Herald* and others, urging him to retract the permit immediately, only for the offending posters, not the ones advertising the event only.

February 19, 1996: Letter to me from the Mayor of Homestead, promising to take opinions into account in the future, but defending their action, citing positive responses for the Grand Prix from the community. He again misses the main point—that even if cigarette companies continue to sponsor the Grand Prix (which should be rethought anyway) our government-owned property is no place for poison messages.

March 1, 2 and 3: The Grand Prix proceeds as planned.

Toward the end of March, just as they did last year, the banners finally come down.

POST-SCRIPT:

February 12, 1997: Article in *Miami Herald* headlined, "'M' is for missing: Grand Prix drops 'Marlboro' from banners."

The article begins: "The M word is gone. After an uproar last year prompted the Florida Department of Transportations to review its policy on roadside advertising, the word "Marlboro" is missing this year from banners on state roads promoting the "Marlboro sponsored Grand Prix of Miami."

There are two pictures shown: one of last year's banners complete with the cigarette logo, the other of this year's. The event only, in yellow and black colors is advertised this year.

February 12, 1997. Letter to editor, which they never publish:

Dear Editor: Thank you for your article, "'M' is for missing," reminding us how an aroused public, with a righteous agenda, can effect beneficial change. Our youth are now safe from the brainwashing of the "poisoned lampposts." I will not mention the tobacco product that is *not* being advertised, since that would give free exposure as you did by publishing the picture of last year's lampposts. And why quote their spokeswoman's assertion that advertising has not been shown to start anyone smoking, only to change brands, without also including in your story how that tired argument has been amply disproved by many well-done medical studies showing just the opposite? Another point to make is that the doom-sayers who threatened that the companies would not sponsor the race again were wrong: there they are, sponsoring the Grand Prix without poisoning our public lampposts. Very truly yours, PG, MD

Taking on city hall, the county and the state can only be worthwhile for one person when the cause is just and when it is ripe, and it requires help from many well intentioned others. We lost both these scrimmages at the time, despite what felt like an all-consuming, valiant fight, sacrificing time away from family and medical practice. By the next year we realized we had won the battle of the poison lampposts by quashing their influence for good. Along with individual patient care, at last we could grasp the significance of the cooperative, larger war against the terrorism of tobacco.

CHAPTER TWENTY-FIVE

Defending "The Complete Physical"

Medicine is, among other things, a detective story. Who dunnit? Which is the guilty organ? Where is the pathology? Why does it hurt? Or—in the case of a healthy, asymptomatic person, where *will* it hurt next? Where are the weak spots? Will the criminal be a recidivist? What intervention will prevent the killer from striking again? Or if a strike is imminent, can we ward it off?

Does it make sense to fragment the crime scene, to examine only one part of the body? To cordon off only those areas where clues have been found before, in other cases, to stick to common entities? To do bean counting of past crimes of other people and to base the investigation on only prior cases, sticking with prior studies and banking on probability? To rush to judgment and make a diagnosis without thorough exploration?

Maybe. But most investigators would seek to delimit the entire crime scene—to do a complete history and physical examination—and to look at each case as unique, systematically, while keeping in mind all they have learned from prior investigations.

But as Family Physicians we restrict ourselves if we talk only about figuring out what illness a sick patient has. So let's look at both the acutely ill patient and the boringly "normal" patient. Let's look at our patient, sitting there in the waiting room—oops, the reception area. What does he have? What could she have? Do we care? If we find it, will intervening make a difference? If we find something for which intervention is not available or desirable, have we hurt him? Do we trust ourselves not to intervene when our intervention will be worse for him than his disease? Or shall we be ostriches, not knowing what's coming?

Prior to this century, nearly all a physician could offer was to tell the patient what he had, how long he had and to give some comfort along the way. (Diagnosis, prognosis, succor.) Now, we teach that if we can't cure the patient we needn't bother to find out what he has. We look only at interventions that are proven. When proof is not produced, we are warned that we could do harm. Faced with uncertainty, the present trend is that we are seldom warned we might do good. Will we do more harm than good? Isn't it a fallacy to teach that because sometimes we overreact with unnecessary anxiety, testing and intervention when we uncover an abnormality, that our patient and we should remain ignorant? What's wrong with all of us learning better and less harmful ways of reacting to the information?

We are exhorted from all sides to look at costs. Does it cost less to do fragmented, specific testing following algorithms based on population screening statistics than to have an experienced physician take a thorough history and perform a physical exam, incorporating the most valid of the screening exams when indicated? Is it worth missing an important screening procedure, having the patient "fall through the cracks" because offices and clinics aren't conducive to extensive review of every chart at episodic visits for sore throats or urinary infections? Are indicators of "quality" and "cost effectiveness" verifiably evaluating the process of patient care, or measuring easily quantifiable entities?

A practice can run smoothly, getting patients in and out quickly, when everyone knows that a periodic (usually yearly) complete assessment visit is advised and adhered to, for the purpose of catching the patient up on all screening, counseling and other missing links in the life of the patient and his or her mental, physical and emotional health.

This should comprise a detailed interview (the history) and a thorough examination (the physical). The interview is a chance to punctuate the patient's narrative with tips and tricks from the physician, regarding indicated changes in life habits and attitudes. Communication on many levels takes place during this dedicated time with the patient. After scrutiny of the entire body, using extensions of our senses such as lights, stethoscopes, magnifiers and other devices, and the taking of specimens, the patient has reason to believe that someone really knows him and cares about him. That is the beginning of trust.

We give a lot of lip service to the development of a doctor-patient relationship, and the fostering of trust. How can a patient trust a doctor who hasn't even examined him? How do you know your patient doesn't have a vulvar carcinoma, just waiting for you to find it? Or a squamous cell carcinoma sitting under a band-aid that she puts on every time she goes to the doctor, because it's "so ugly" and she's embarrassed. (A true case). Or painless hematuria which heralds a renal cell carcinoma?

At least the trajectories of colon cancer, hypercholesterolemia, hypertension and diabetes are proven now. But what about before the proof? Was that a reason not to look? Not to test? Not to measure? The usual impetus to earlier screening for preventable disease is to have had enough patients die for the physician to realize that if only he/she had just looked for the disease, it could have been found earlier—and cured—or at least ameliorated. If anyone should be doing complete assessments, it is the generalist.

Although we often lose our patients to specialists who know more about their special disease, we are the ones to whom the patient first presents. Unfortunately, large, randomized trials are not the way to uncover anything useful about rare or uncommon events, and many of our patients have rare or uncommon entities.

One of the most misleading maxims in medicine is that common things occur commonly, that if you hear hoof beats outside, it's horses, not zebras. Although both are quite true, it is also true that rare diseases occur commonly—because there are so many of them. Within everyone's practice—but only if you look—there will be your share of really strange and fascinating zebras. You won't have the same ones as your colleague (each one is not that common), but you'll have them. The patients can't help it that their disease is uncommon or rare, but they're every bit as sick with it as those with common entities.

You will not find these diseases or conditions until they're so obvious, they scream at you—unless you look. This does not mean indiscriminate testing of everybody for everything. That is what paramedical people would have to do, since they have not been trained even to know the names of most of the rarer entities. We needn't restrict this concept to disease entities; we can talk about atypical management problems, such as medication reactions, psychosocial interactions, stress reactions, physical training idiosyncrasies. But that's what being a physician is about—taking care of everyone, in the most appropriate way, and knowing what is going on with that patient. There is no other way than to examine the patient. One of my professors used to say, "Listen to the patient; he's telling you the diagnosis." I might add to that, "Look at (examine) the patient—with all your skills—he's giving the solution to your medical mystery story."

CHAPTER TWENTY-SIX

Crossing the Line

When discussing a fringe treatment, diet book, or borderline practitioner with a patient, my response used to be, "We in medicine are different from others who want to sell you something." I used to explain that expertise and wisdom are a physician's only stock in trade. I would emphasize that we are professionals, not celery-tonic hawkers who profit by what we recommend.

Physicians might tell their patients that a given product could help them, but we would never try to sell it to them. That would be a clear conflict. I would explain that we might package a product and make it available at near cost, if no pharmacy or drugstore is nearby. But our opinion about a drug or nutritional supplement should never be colored by our ability to earn more income by selling it.

The patient usually responded with a greater understanding of the difference between physicians and the commercial world. But these days I can no longer say this to patients. Why? Because many in our community have begun to sell both drugs and "nutritionals." Where does this salesmanship stop? What about tissues? How about toilet paper? After all, a clean nose is a public health benefit, as is a clean rear.

It's an icy incline. By such logic almost anything can be justified. The quest for short-term gain by a few physicians can erode the integrity of the whole profession. Yet most of us are too chicken to criticize or confront such physicians. That's why we should support resolutions that affirm general principles that professionals should follow. When the American Medical Association's House of Delegates endorsed the position that no profit should be made from selling health-related products in the office, it reflected the sense and sensibility of most physicians. The AMA is not always right, but this time it is "right as rain"—no matter how many of us are jumping on the bandwagon of in-office retailing.

We need to admit that physicians are humble humans whose impartiality about treatments can be affected by monetary gain. We should avoid putting ourselves in a questionable position that blurs the line between what we recommend and where the patient buys it.

What do I tell patients now? As a libertarian, I tell them it's a free country and people have a right to do as they please. But I also point out that we and our patients are free to change our opinions of physicians if we believe that they have crossed an ethical line. If some of us want to sell nutritionals, that's fine, as long as we don't use our MD degrees and our relationships with patients to further that goal. We shouldn't pretend that reading a company's promotional material is continuing medical education. And if we leave the MD after our names, we shouldn't expect it to enhance trust with patients or fellow physicians.

But if we want to earn the respect and credibility of our colleagues and patients, we will study nutrition because it's enlightening. Many doctors have done this for years because they can't take care of patients otherwise. I have friends in certain specialties who never learned much about total health and nutrition because there was nothing to be gained from it. Now, all of a sudden, they're experts on the topic, because now they're selling a product.

Let's offer our advice, write our prescriptions, and send our patients to the stores to buy what we recommend. It will take a critical mass of physicians to stand up to the wave of self-defeating commercialism in our bottom-line culture. If we can't practice as professionals, perhaps we should leave the profession. Perhaps some of us already have.

CHAPTER TWENTY-SEVEN

Summit Solutions: The Medical Doctor's Role

We physicians caring for patients seldom control the design, research and implementation of entire medical systems in our own region, country or hemisphere. Yet the prevailing winds of medicine profoundly affect conditions under which we are privileged to provide medical care. Although we are usually swept by tides, we are often said to be making the weather; the deficiencies of various systems may be ascribed to a perception that the "medical profession" with its treatment orientation is dominating public health policy.

Medical care is the least significant of the basic triad of public health which consists of prevention, medical care, and rehabilitation. Data supports the observation that equity in medical care fails to assure equity in health. (In England and Wales, the inequality in mortality of social classes has actually widened since the establishment of the National Health Service, and in Canada in the late '70s, despite their system, the difference in disability-free life-expectancy between the lowest and highest social classes was eleven years.)[1]

A wider gap between rich and poor paradoxically does not mean worsening conditions for the poor. Where this has been well-studied (England) real health of the poorest improves, while the relative difference widens.[2] If our sense of justice demands equality, we are discomfited. It may be a small price to pay, though—allowing the rich to get richer and the healthy healthier—if by so doing, the unhealthy become healthier in tandem.[3]

Those who organize society can offer only the justice of equality of opportunity; the rest is up to the people themselves. The idea of "free" medical care is born out of the compassionate desire to take good care of people. We feel embarrassment when someone sick goes without care because of bad luck or catastrophe. Yet the ultimate caring is inherent in allowing people to take care of themselves, whenever they can.

Some paternalistically believe that people cannot or will not take care of themselves; therefore, central planning is required, either by government or big business. This does not give people credit for understanding their own best interests. For free people to act responsibly, they must obtain a background of excellent health education, provided by television and other educational mass technology that motivates towards healthy behaviors and choices.

More funding directed into appropriate public-health-intensive efforts can be targeted in psychologically valid ways to affect the segments of the population shown to be most in need of each message. Patients who, in spite of education, are unable or refuse to care for themselves can go to publicly funded health clinics. It will be clear that to afford better one must work harder and save, but there will still be that "safety net."

Efforts to train more generalists and to improve prevention should not impede innovation, which is the nurture of the future. Innovation can occur not just in developed countries. Progress depends on optimism and high levels of research and development in all specialties, in medicine and other societal technologies.

Health and development overlap daily in new ways, yet new methods mean little if they do not reach people.[4] Even in a perfect system, people get sick, prevention fails, illnesses develop. The doctor comes, first to diagnose, then to alleviate, sometimes to cure, always to comfort. Although physicians may find niches in clinics and hospitals, many will prefer independence and entrepreneurial spirit, usually more for issues of control than income.

It is to the benefit of the public that the medical world stays safe for diversity. Patients should be able to choose from a wide range of qualified practitioners. Each physician defines—within the range of accepted medical practice—his/her own vision of what excellent medical care to an individual patient can be. Patient guidelines for screening and treatment—apart from becoming rapidly out-dated—may be suitable for large-scale populations, when taxes and/or insurance health plans eager to save (make) money pay for care. These "cookbooks" may differ from recommendations for individual patients.

Medicine will always be an art.[5] Each situation is different. Many persons with extra income prefer to exchange their own dollars for superior medical care rather than for foreign travel, consumer goods or luxuries. (More procedures are not necessarily better, but more time with patients and more care in diagnosis and follow-up is usually better and cannot be afforded on a bare-bones budget or on capitation plans.)

Planners may forget that the source of all funds is the people, themselves. In well-meaning efforts to lower costs and overuse/abuse they seek to control the people's resources. This is not taking from the advantaged to redistribute. This is taking the patients' own money, skimming some off, giving only some of it back. Then they bestow "free" medical care. They usually mandate which doctors to see, and oversee all arrangements, while diminishing physicians' power to advocate for patients.

Letting patients keep the original resource (their money, the fruit of their labor) will allow them to spend where and when they want, without the interference of third parties. Favorable laws (tax-exempt Medical Savings Accounts and portable insurance) would make this practical and affordable for patients. Physicians bemoan the loss of the doctor-patient relationship, as they lose control of their own profession. Many people, doctors and patients, may be hurt before the pendulum swings back to that personal encounter at the bedside.

Free patients will choose free doctors who will care about and for them, charge them a reasonable price, encourage preventive care, and advise buying good insurance for the infrequent accident or illness. Apart from overseeing the medical profession's own enforcement of medical standards and credentialing, and making insurance available, third party micromanagement will prove to increase costs, to skew incentives and to deflect attention from healing.

The public's health directly affects the type of cases all practicing physicians will see. Prevention and rehabilitation efforts by planners need intensification and support. Cities and countries with large numbers of poor people may need public clinics for some time. Attempts to control total medical care—by government or big business—may bring potentially self-sufficient patients and doctors downward into systems that divert resources on the way to providing average or mediocre medical care. Rather, the goal should be to maintain freedom and independence for doctors and patients leading to superior, affordable medical attention for all.

Endnotes

1   Terris, Milton; The health situation in the Americas, in International Health, a North South Debate, Human Resources Development No. 95, Pan American Health Organization (PAHO). 1992. p.77—85.

2   Townsend, P; Davidson; N; Whitehead, M.; The Black report and the health divide. Harmondsworth: Penguin, 1992.

3   Charlton, BG.; Is inequality bad for the national health? Lancet 1994. Jan 22: 221.

4   Guerra de Macedo, C; The great challenges of the nineties and their impact on international health, in International Health, a North South Debate, PAHO, 1992, p. 1—5.

5   Contandriopoulos, AP; Cost and equity of health systems, in International Health, a North South Debate, PAHO, 1992, p. 87—101.

CHAPTER TWENTY-EIGHT

Speaking Out: Growing a Tasteless Tomato

A sense of desperation, possibly undeserved, pervades the American health care scene, leading to various attempts to remedy what appears to some to be a floundering non-system, incapable of serving 37 million people who are said to be without health insurance.

Yet those of us who actually take care of patients on the front lines know that we are still caring for sick— and well—people and accepting whatever payment we get. Often, we accept no payment yet continue to render care.

There are many causes of the medical chaos that is perceived today. For physicians and patients both, the most severe impact involves the diversion of the art of healing into business and administrative efforts. These tasks involve maintaining armies of administrators, insurance workers, and attorneys. Some of these are our own physicians, persuaded that their efforts should be so diverted, and paid more for their new directions than for providing patient care.

The ultimate health care dollar becomes split among layers of intermediaries; we are no longer buying tomatoes directly from the farmer. No wonder they have become so expensive and so tasteless.

The question of how to attain universal access to medical care while preserving the best features of our current system usually invokes plans for gaining control of runaway costs—a laudable goal. Many people take the simplistic approach that central planning, in the form of universal health insurance, will solve all problems.

But central planning and control will more likely be counterproductive. Why? Because they do not permit true freedom for both doctors and patients, nor give room for the additive, incremental, and catholic nature of medical progress. Not all chaos is bad, as modern theories of chaos indicate.

A distinction between optimal care and minimal, acceptable care needs to be made. The knotty problems of access to care and of restraint without rationing could be solved by:

- A basic floor of care that includes preventive care offered to everyone and funded through existing or new mechanisms, based on ability to pay. This would be a minimalist approach, including only those interventions and screening tests that yield proven reductions in the rate of illness and death and can be proven cost-effective.

- A comprehensive approach, through which in-depth examination, preventive measures, treatment (some of which might be on the cutting edge of progress and not yet proven), and counseling are purchased based on the true worth of those services given by physicians able to offer such care to patients eager to purchase it.

Ongoing, predictable expenses—yes, even mammograms—are made more costly by funneling funds through government or insurance agencies before getting them to the people who actually do the work. Both doctors and patients need to see this obvious point. Insurance should be for illness, thereby spreading true risk. Incentives, but not payment, should be built in for preventive care over and above the basic floor.

Public health education and advertising should be expanded to make health a popular habit. If payment is the only obstacle, other public or private funding, but not insurance, should be triggered. How much of the recent increases in insurance premiums is due to each specialty wanting its particular activity to be covered?

Medical care to maximize health is not universally valued. Many patients won't accept care even when sick, while others "overutilize." Differing attitudes should be free to flourish. With the system proposed here, the best features of our present, individualistic approach would be preserved even as no one would go without a basic level of adequate care. Those who put health care high on their priority list will budget or insure for it as they currently do for other, less important items for which they pay willingly.

CHAPTER TWENTY-NINE

Home Free: Safe for Now

We can rejoice that the country is safe from a federally-imposed "health care system."

However, corporate machinations are doing what we feared government would do: wrest the medical profession out of our hands, replacing medical judgment with administrative layering, while renaming it "access, quality and cost-containment." Some physicians are so frustrated by the disarray that they have succumbed to the notion that a single-payer federal system would now be an improvement!

There Is Access

The canard that we are the only industrialized country without guaranteed health care belies the actual medical care our citizens receive. Although we don't carry a one-size-fits-all card, this does not mean we are not "universally covered." It also ignores the inferior type of care in many countries said to provide access. Most of us have treated foreign patients. We know the level of their education and sophistication. We hear eye-witness accounts of how they are examined and treated (or not treated).

Here in the United States, no one is denied care. We do not see people dying on the streets unless they have refused help. A breakdown in the system provokes outcries, for we have come to expect near perfection. When the county hospital here missed one breast cancer that went too far and "fell through the cracks" of the system, the whole community was outraged, and steps were taken immediately to correct the situation. Was that because our system was so bad? No—it was because it was so good.

Our expectations were that such a thing would not and could not occur. By our peculiar response to error was our high standard defined.

Cost Concerns

President Clinton said it outright on national television at the outset of his campaign for "health care reform." He said yes, we all had access. But at what price? He stressed that the poor were mainly getting their care in the emergency rooms (ERs) of the cities, using those departments as clinics at all hours, at great expense.

The expense is not to the poor patients, but to the rest of us. We can't disagree with these observations. Either way, the expense would be to the rest of us, through higher taxes, or higher insurance premiums to pay for spreading the risk of the least healthy, or through using ERs instead of neighborhood clinics.

Sometimes their poor health is through their own poor decisions, because circumstances close out true choice. The HMOs and insurance companies have carefully cherry-picked the healthiest, and use "rationing" (perverse incentives to doctors) by which to by-pass care for the neediest. Even when the poor have a physician willing to care for them, they still tend to use the ER because that's where the action is, where their friends go, and where they define sociologically their places in the medical system. Ingrained habits are hard to change.

Regardless of most cost-efficient venue, sick people are being taken care of in offices and ERs, whether they pay or not. We do have access, and could have cost control, right now.

Patients' Own Money: Laws to Enable

There is more than one way to be "covered." It doesn't have to be insurance or health plans. Insurance makes sense only to spread risk for unexpected care. Regular medical care can be paid directly by all but the poorest, using dollars saved by an educated populace. If laws are passed which allow tax saving for those dollars, as well as savings for long-term care in later years, patients will be able to make their own rational plans. Insurance is the most expensive way to pay for ordinary medical care, since it filters original dollars through non-medical persons first, losing value as those dollars are skimmed. When people spend their own money they will educate themselves as to what is good health. The total amount spent on unnecessary care will decline. People would pay attention to public-health messages, which would be a proper function of government and the media, and are conspicuously lacking now.

Formulas For Failure

Much of what is happening today in medicine seems unconscionable. Not everyone goes along. Just because it's a steam roller doesn't make it durable. Some of the highest flyers may be in for the biggest falls. Mergers and acquisitions may be signs of desperation rather than strength. There may come a time when "capitation" will be considered not only unethical and immoral, but illegal, because of injustices to patients and doctors alike. Why? Because it purveys an impossible contract between a doctor and a patient, which the doctor cannot possibly honor properly.

Cursory Care

With capitation, the doctor receives a set amount of money per month for each patient. He/she bets the patients won't all "collect" on his/her promise to take care of them. The bet is that many will never call, many will not get sick. If the patients were to be aggressively educated they would seek preventive care. But the bet is that most won't, for there would no be time to give careful physical exams to all of them. Yet, because they pay very little or nothing, many will come in for the least little thing that bothers them, not realizing most of the money they've paid into their plans has gone to administrators and company profit—and not to the doctors and nurses. So the offices are full of people who don't need to be there, receiving rushed, focused, episodic care, even as the doctor resists his/her previous tendency to encourage periodic well-patient visits for thoughtful preventive care. Then, if they all get sick at once, the doctor is really strapped, and won't be able to function or "afford" the arrangement. The medical management magazines are full of articles warning doctors that they might not be able to "afford" capitation. What they really mean is that only those who best develop systems to give cursory care can manage it without running ragged or going out of business. That is the reason capitation is immoral for its effect on patients.

"Risk" Of Good Doctoring

The concept of business risk has no place in this profession, even though it is a watchword of antitrust and commerce. Physicians took enough risk dedicating eight years to schooling, another three to five to residency, including nights, weekends, with abrogation of family life and all else. Opening an office and keeping constantly current is risky enough. No one should have to "risk" becoming an insurance company for unpredictable illness of people we think we're forced to care for. We are not insurance companies. Standing ready to "sell" our hours of service and our expertise is quite enough. That is the reason capitation is immoral for its effect on doctors.

Hidden Agendas

There may come a time when contracts which are "normal" now will become unethical, immoral and illegal. These contracts muzzle the doctor and his/her staff from leveling with patients and telling them what perverse incentives are built into the plans and contracts they, the doctors, have signed. The unwitting patient believes in the tacit agreement that has prevailed in the history of medicine until now: that a doctor will first keep faith with his/her patient. What they aren't told is that the doctor must keep faith with the contract, and is in an impossible position. These contracts chance personal and financial ruin, or even legal action and incarceration, should the doctor or any staff member breach confidentiality of their terms. The patient ought to know the terms of any contracts that affect the doctor's relationships. This is the basis of the ama's Patient Choice platform, which calls for the right to full disclosure.

Medical Care, Not Health Care

Let's discuss medical care, not health care. Society, teachers, advertisers, public health persons, the media and the government can go far in contributing to the well-being of the population by helping to make healthy habits routine, and by keeping life-style and social issues constantly in the public eye. Educational functions can be performed by others (in my office they are). But each patient has a learning curve and a readiness for certain information. To come up with the very thing they need to direct their behavior into healthier choices is part of the art and persuasion of medicine. It carries the timing and authority of the person who has just carefully examined that patient. Advice coming at that special time must be more impressive in the patient's eyes, and therefore more effective. That is part of our mission, and why "laying on of hands" means so much. However, our function—what we can do that no one else can—is to figure out why patients feel sick, and to strike preemptively at hidden pathology which we uncover. We function as doctors when people become ill; one might say that our training is somewhat wasted on well people, except that we are constantly finding things wrong or improvable with nearly every patient, if we take the time to look.

Whose Expertise?

Citizens can give support to research in medicine and basic science, but only physicians will be in the examining rooms, reliably verifying diagnoses made by physician-extenders, deciding which treatments apply to which patients, evaluating and chancing new treatments, and dancing along the undulating wave of future cures. Only physicians can be trusted with this daunting combination of responsibilities.

The training and experience of legislators, administrators, corporate ceos, assistants and other practitioners is neither broad nor current enough, nor have they been strained through the colander of hairy nights in the hospitals, and days in the clinics. Making, shouldering and living with the final decisions falls to the doctor.

Continuity of care in individual patients is not just a buzzword or a marketing ploy. The filtering of new information and putting it to use, though aided by mathematicians, statisticians, pharmacologists and researchers, still requires that final common pathway: the physicians.

Free Doctors, Free Patients

Any valid cost curbs must be shunted into better patient care, and more direct control and autonomy in the sunshine, for doctor and patient. Better bottom lines for other entities, including government, business, or the doctor, him/herself, are not the goal. There is nothing wrong with making a reasonable living. There is nothing wrong with commercial activity. But a profession differs significantly from a business, and the onus is on us to bear that standard relentlessly. Those who doubt that difference will find it out to their dismay, when too sick and weak to protest. Our medical care system—whatever changes it undergoes, and whatever legislative burdens are added or removed—must always maintain the integrity of the physician and his/her ability to function independently, influenced only by autonomous patients, not commercial or governmental organizations with non-medical agendas.

CHAPTER THIRTY

The Mercy Merger

This is the story as it happened, strictly from my viewpoint.

I was sitting in the doctor's dining room at South Miami Hospital, happily having lunch with some of my colleagues, when one, a cardiologist, said to me, "You know we have to do something about this. They're going through with it—it's a done deal. There must be something that can be done. You are the one who got that terrible malpractice law repealed (he was referring to the march to Tallahassee), surely you could do something." He sounded serious and desperate.

"Yeah, there ought to be something done," some of the other doctors chimed in.

"I have no idea what you're talking about," I said. I had been out of the loop of hospital politics for a while.

They said incredulously, "You haven't heard about the Mercy merger?"

"No," I said. "Tell me."

They went on to recount the news that the large Catholic hospital, Mercy Hospital, was about to sign a merger agreement with Baptist Health Systems, the umbrella organization for Baptist Hospital and South Miami Hospital. (Since then, there are three more hospitals owned by Baptist Health). They were doing this for business reasons, but, according to my concerned informants, there were major other considerations.

I said, "Okay—all of you have known this. Why tell me this now? I'm sure if there were something that could be done it would have been done by now, or it will be done by someone else. You certainly don't need me."

"No one is doing a thing," they said. "No one can think of anything. We have no power. The doctors are helpless in the grip of the Hospital. They do what they want."

With that, I began to be a bit interested. I have always thought a hospital existed as a place for doctors (the only ones who really know what to do for sick people) to bring their patients—not an entity existing for its own growth and aggrandizement, using patients as a shield.

"So what, as you see it, are the implications if the merger goes through?" I asked. The cardiologist looked at me as though I were mentally challenged.

"Don't you get it?" he asked.

"Not entirely," I answered. "Tell me."

He proceeded to enumerate the effects a Catholic hospital would have on practices at Baptist Health Hospitals, including our main one, South Miami Hospital. He said that now, abortion was between a woman and her physician. It would be completely outlawed—in all cases, even that of anencephaly (where an infant has no brain and will surely die if allowed to go to term and be delivered). He said that ordinary birth control advice about methods and certainly birth control pills would be banned, as would tubal ligation; that even discussing matters not approved by the Catholic Church's rigorous and strictest doctrines would be banned. He said that all Catholic beliefs would have to be imposed on the entire system.

At the time, I doubted his assertions. I would later find out, from an organization called, Catholics for a Free Choice, that he was absolutely right. I asked him if the board of the hospital had taken leave of their senses. He said he just assumed they didn't think women were that important to them; that the business angle was the driving force. He said there was no one to speak up for what was clearly right for our hospital and our people. I took this whole conversation to mean that he expected me to pull some rabbit out of a hat. After all, a done deal is a done deal—but that was his point. Someone needed to do something and no one had. So he plopped the whole thing down in my lap.

I could have walked away. I could have said, "Well, if it's not important enough to anyone else, why should I care?" knowing that to care about this would set off a whole string of obligations, need for creative thought, plotting and planning, and organizing lots of other people. This would be like so many other causes—a concerted, consuming effort. To think otherwise would be delusional. I left the doctor's dining room telling them that I would think about it, and I went back to my busy family practice office. That night, I agonized over whether I should get involved in this. Knowing myself I realized how passionate I could get, how single-minded, how preoccupied. I knew it would be a huge time and emotional commitment. Then I began to reflect on what it would really mean for the women of our County.

The fact was that the Baptist Health System had essentially taken over the southern part of Miami-Dade County, and was becoming a behemoth. We did not know then that it would swallow Doctors Hospital, Homestead Hospital, and Mariner's Hospital. I reflected on what those Catholic restrictions, cited by my friend, would mean to all the women subsumed by the territory then covered by just Baptist Hospital and South Miami Hospital. I began to imagine that I was one of those women (which I was, but no longer of child-bearing age at the time), who would need a service acceptable to me and my doctor, but not to the restrictive, Catholic rule-makers running the hospital. What a colossal injustice that would be! That creative imagination is what sucked me into deciding that I would do it. Once I made that decision, failure became no option. I would have to do whatever it took.

I honestly didn't really believe all I had heard. In 1997, the internet was not as convenient as it is now, but you could do quite a lot. I found an organization called Catholics for a Free Choice.[1] In their archives, they still have salient articles written around that time, warning that mergers of Catholic with non-Catholic hospitals were dangerous to women's reproductive health, and, after the facts recounted here, a specific reference to a physician at South Miami Hospital who called a meeting of the entire hospital staff, who voted, almost unanimously, to block the change in the abortion policy and then to block the merger itself.

---

1   Then, their website was "catholics4choice.org," and now it is "catholicsforchoice.org."

I was that physician. Although I hadn't personally called that meeting—I asked for time to speak at a general, hospital medical staff meeting.

Here is how it unfolded. I became thoroughly knowledgeable about the issue. Catholics for a Free Choice did a great job in educating me. They completely corroborated all that my friend had told me about what happens when Catholic hospitals merge with regular hospitals. They insist on their own restrictive rules—or it's no deal. Their organization was already dealing with this issue and could cite numerous instances of successful activist goals being achieved, meaning they succeeded in supporting those trying to kill such deals. They provided a service called MergerWatch, whereby they listed all the activity in the whole country, state by state. They looked upon these attempted mergers as a concerted effort of the church to impose their restrictive ideas all over the country, unbeknownst to the rest of us. They looked at their organization as performing a crucial service of alerting doctors and patients to this unfair and unwise subversion. I was shocked that such an organization could exist, untrammeled by the church itself, but very encouraged that these progressive Catholics were fighting such valiant battles.

I taught myself PowerPoint in the heat of the battle. I had to, even though it took hours. I learned to insert things like clip art into printed slides to make my points hit home. I reasoned that I had to make a convincing appeal to the doctors to rise up and exert the real power that they had.

I asked for only four minutes of time to give a presentation to the medical staff at an upcoming meeting, assuming they would not give me more. The Baptist Health System, of which "our" hospital, South Miami Hospital, was one part, held all the cards and all the power, and could direct the meetings the way they wanted them to go. They granted my request for the four minutes. I don't think they had any idea of the persuasive nature of the logic I would present, with slides to emphasize the points, and that at the end of the presentation I would ask the doctors to vote then and there as to their position on whether reproductive rights were between a woman and her physician, within existing laws of this country, or should be allowed to be governed by religious convictions imposed by a hospital board at which the doctors themselves had no significant input.

The point of the presentation was that a hospital is nothing without its doctors. It is bricks and mortar. The doctors feel defeated, powerless in the face of big money and influence beyond the control of any one of us. But together, we have all the power, even though we are not a formal union. They cannot exist without us. We have only to understand that and exert that power, when it becomes necessary and right. We could start, not by withholding medical care (which would be punitive to patients and to ourselves), but by refusing to participate in any committees (without which the hospital could lose its accreditation) and exerting other forms of collective action to achieve the goal of persuading the hospital that it does not want to go against the will of its doctors. But what was the will of the doctors?

Bear in mind that, although much of the medical staff was latin (mainly Cuban, but also others) and Catholic themselves, they were physicians, knowledgeable of where human and women's rights become privacy rights between a woman and her physician. Whether they were personally for or against abortion, itself, all but two physicians in the entire group of over three hundred present that night voted to preserve the patient doctor relationship, and the right to abortion that had existed before the board changed it (abortion permitted if a woman's health was threatened, versus only if her life was threatened), as well as all other reproductive rights.

Meanwhile, we were simultaneously contacting women known to be activists in the community. But not just women were interested. Men too had a stake in this outcome. We called a meeting at one of the synagogues, another at one of the churches; we had meetings at the home of a husband and wife doctor couple, who were good friends of mine, who were extremely active and supportive, and helped coordinate everything. This doctor couple were crucial to the whole effort. Many of the meetings were held at their house. I found out much later that they had been instrumental in setting the stage, behind the scenes, in multiple hospital task forces and committees, for the success of all that happened subsequently.

We developed a core group of physicians, and one of community members, that even included some members of the Florida legislature. The message was always the same. Women's reproductive rights and the right of the patient-doctor free relationship came first, and could not coexist with restrictive policies.

I became so personally involved in all these meetings and coordinating everything that I barely had time for my family and my medical practice. I was careful to be very inclusive to anyone who wanted to participate, and to spread the credit around to everyone, since, in truth, it became a classic study in grass-roots activism. We got quite a bit of press coverage, even without asking for it. The American Civil Liberties Union got involved. There were lawyers waiting in the wings, ready for civil action and lawsuits, should they persist in going ahead with the merger.

Suddenly, the "done deal" was done for. We killed it. They gave up. Working together we prevailed. And our hospital (and the entire Baptist Health System Hospitals now and in the future), its doctors and its women, were safe and free again.

CHAPTER THIRTY-ONE

The Eyes of Our Patients: The Most Telling of All LCDs

How to Make Things Better

Why aren't things better?

First, who says things aren't better? True, we must address our failures, but what about our successes? When considering mistakes and errors, consider the denominator. How many wrong turns (numerator) over how many right ones (denominator)? Or how many total turns (the real denominator)? Only those who do nothing make no mistakes. Articles in the lay press, discussing the second careers of the elderly, brag about how young seventy is these days. They tout the advanced management of diabetes, coronary artery disease, infectious diseases and other causes of death and disability, all of which are managed by today's physicians, who are the chief engineers of these patients' wellbeing and long life.

Yet we bewail that things are not better. The perception of poor quality seems to shine out from the backdrop of such high expectations. The idea that we have lost what was good seems to have come with the bigness boom and the "techie" touch. The bigger the group, the more lost in the crowd are the hapless patients. And now the fixers of such problems would have us become bigger and more technical, as though that will automatically change things for the better.

The groupthink these days is "systems," a way of avoiding individual responsibility and diffusing/defusing the pointed finger. This keeps the lawyers (a huge part of the problem of poor quality—remember autopsies?

Remember real learning from our mistakes?) at bay. This also creates business for the makers and managers of "systems."

To be sure, systems are very important, but they are neither the whole nor even the main story. The computer is only one of the useful tools for our work. Yet we have come so far as a federally backed mandate for universal EMRS.

I'm no tech dinosaur. I had a privately designed office billing system on a twenty-five pound Kaypro with a CPM operating system back in 1984. I was an "early adopter," the "first on my block." We do electronic filing now. But I no more think everyone having an EMR will change what ails us than I think snowmobiles have improved Yellowstone.

Sadly, more data, more quickly accessible, could deter us from looking into the eyes of our patients, the most telling of all LCDS.

This brings us to the well-known, influential, physician businessman (not clinician), whose righteous indignation over his own travails in the maze of medicine, so impressed reporters of the *Wall Street Journal* and *Boston Globe*, in addition to editorialist John H. Wasson, MD, that his personal opinions have been given elevated status and circulation. Complaining about his wife's poor treatment when she was lost medically and emotionally, in the maze of a large, impersonal organization, he then— from the lofty perch of his own large organization—recommended that we all subject ourselves to even larger and more impersonal organizational schemes, in the name of efficiency, cost saving and "quality."

Could not the reverse be true? We have become disconnected from our real doctors, our family/generalist physicians, by subspecialists doing not only their own jobs, but preempting the generalists' purview. The patient needs coordination of care, hiring and firing these very subspecialists by someone qualified to oversee their performance close at hand.

Insurance companies ("health plans") and hospitals have wrested power away from all but the most tenacious personal physicians to develop systems that effectively disincentivize them by excluding them systematically from the care of the sickest patients and interrupting continuity of care. This takes away the patients' most important link and advocate.

Our graduating residents are acculturated to accept fragmented care and handing their sickest patients over to hospitalists.

In fact, it has been "systems" that have "done us in." Had this physician's wife been my patient, my name would have been on her hospital bracelet, from admission to discharge. I would have willingly taken responsibility for her total care, including negotiating the puzzling patchwork that is today's mega-hospital. All the subspecialists who write orders would have their orders checked through me, not to countermand them, but to coordinate them. Any family member, husband included, would be able to call me at any time for questions or solace, since, as a family doctor, I'm available and trained in all branches of medicine and psychiatry, in breadth, if not in depth. I would have known full well that she was a lawyer, since I would have been the thread of continuity throughout her life for as long as she was my patient, and even if she were a new patient. The question of how this type of coordinated care is reimbursed would take more discussion, but is irrelevant, since in the end, it saves—not costs—resources, not to mention lives and psyches.

Far from being banned from the ICUs (Intensive Care Units), the family doctor should be called into ICUs as a consultant, for any patients who have the misfortune of being taken care of by subspecialists only. As expert and indispensable as these specialists are, they are immersed in one field, dependent on nurses, who are wonderful but are not generalist physicians, to be the equivalent of the generalist, spotting conditions outside of the particular specialists' purviews. Sadly, his very own sick wife got lost and mismanaged in the bowels of a large hospital system. The makeup of such systems guarantees that there will be snafus, right and left.

If one wanted to design systems where errors would multiply, they couldn't do better than our mega hospitals or even our large medical groups. I like the way the call for self awareness article suggests that not systems, but individuals and their way of thinking, feeling and behaving could be changed to prevent errors.

The unfamiliar definitions sound a strangely familiar note: "refining physicians' emotional and cognitive capacities," sounds an awful lot like what we used to call "caring." The error of giving low-level decision making attention, rather than seeing all possibilities, sounds an awful lot like getting rid of the patient's problems the quickest way possible.

Can it be that we have begun to pick the wrong people to be our doctors? That intellectual capacity is not the only attribute? That the innate caring—the person with heart—is not as common among our ranks as they used to be or should be?

In the call for "systems," where is the personal investment? It is distanced, the less the "system" is our own—more evidence that large systems are counterproductive. Those of us in private practice have our own systems. Some of us have sought to teach those that work to others, and to encourage small units of systems that are nimble on their feet, and can change to meet new technology and new evidence.

Ideas such as group visits have their place, especially for chronic disease management, as an adjunct to the usual doctor-patient interactions. But these visits are useless in picking up subtle or even blatant changes in individual patients' conditions that cannot be measured by a canned laboratory test within an automatic protocol.

Nothing supplants, or can supplant, the face-to-face relationship between a doctor and patient, just as there is no substitute for the nuclear family, a father, mother and children. There are orphanages and group homes that do a creditable job, but they'll always be second best.

Bigger is not better. Small and personal is good: one doctor, one patient, one at a time, with specialists coming and going as needed. It is not the lack of systems, but of individuals imbued with concerted efforts to revert to the first principles of medicine.

The concept of small and personal completely assuages patients' dissatisfactions, and leads to fewer errors, better communication and more real caring. That's how to make things better.

CHAPTER THIRTY-TWO

Health "Reform"—Mistaken Conclusions

"O say does that star spangled banner yet wave, O'er the land of the free and the home of the brave!" Conclusions that central planning to achieve "universal health care" will advance the people's and the doctors' causes are mistaken. We who believe it won't happen that way are just as "well-meaning" in our defense of freedom and individual rights for doctor and patient believing that ultimate progress and satisfaction lies with freedom, in medicine as in life.

Universal medical care for all can be achieved without the central planning/central payer schemes that attempt to solve the problem. Other countries that seem to have better care, with more socialized systems, are fraught with problems, different but equal in impact to ours. Some have systems from which we can learn, and we should. Until we, ourselves and our leaders, finally confront our own shortcomings (our lack of education while young and healthy for medical contingency and our willingness to value and pay for it ourselves, up front) we physicians and our patients will suffer and struggle.

The idea that medical care should be free is strange. Someone must pay. We all pay anyway, one way or another. We must be compassionate as a society and pay for unfortunates who can't or won't pull their own weight. But the rest of us can and should take care of ourselves, as we do for food, housing, recreation, cosmetics, alcohol, etc. We should be tired of the equation, Insurance = medical care. We have seen how managed care "insurance" has mangled our care and frustrated our doctors. My fellow physicians and I give care, with or without "insurance." (Yes, we do need to be paid.) Doctor = medical care = real equation.

The true equations:

Insurance = expensive care

Insurance = hospital care

Insurance = skims dollars off every encounter for commerce/government

Insurance = necessary—to spread UNLIKELY risk.

Insurance = too expensive for known, expected costs (oil, gas, well care, even mammograms—because they are predictable and cheaper if NOT paid with insurance)

If you pay your doctor directly, you get more for your dollar.

If you pay your doctor via insurance, you are also paying for the insurance company's or the hospital's or the government's buildings, executives, secretaries, slick advertising, computers, paper and much more. And it's likely your doctor is not free to do what he/she thinks is best, but what the insurance company demands, because they are in business to make money, not in a profession to render service. And, if you don't get sick, you have given up your money for nothing.

You should keep that money for yourself.

This is why Health Savings Accounts make so much sense. Apart from allowing you to keep your own money and spend it wisely where you choose, these accounts lead to accountability in "the system" by making sure everyone has catastrophic insurance (which is what insurance was supposed to be, not first dollar coverage). Of course, the indigent population would still need clinics run by local or federal government agencies. But 85% or more of the population can and should have their own Health Savings Accounts, and then go shopping for the doctors who give them the best care for their buck.

Please keep these concepts in the forefront of your mind, when thinking about all the recent talk on health systems.

CHAPTER THIRTY-THREE

Disillusioned or Enlightened—
The Choices of Free Doctors and Patients

Dear Editor, FPReport:

I read with sadness the letter from the disillusioned medical student, juxtaposed with your June, 2003 cover story, "Family medicine leaders foretell future of the specialty, US Health system," because I visualized part of this story fifteen years ago, when I published a warning we should have heeded then, when HMOS were the bandwagon of the day.[1] Your article echoes my predictions, vindicating my choice to be "a dinosaur" (not in technology, but in practice style), staying solo, while my colleagues got burned and their patients scorched, as groups formed and fell. So—the HMO house of cards came tumbling down. Now, we're looking for a brave new world again. As long as our leaders have ambition to pour us into some controllable mold, we will not achieve our destiny as family doctors. Our leadership could foster, for our patients and us, individual freedom and autonomy to avoid being doomed between the Scylla of the state and the Charybdis of commerce. Isn't it time to see the AAFP defend the individual practitioner and patient, rather than looking for ways of homogenizing the process and the people? Isn't it time to keep our specialty safe for the diversity we all talk about?

Just as we are free citizens in this country, we must remain free patients and doctors—not hostages—in our medical care. Rich or poor, not everyone values his/her health equally. Those who do should not be forced into a mediocre, one-size-fits-all medical model. It is a compliment, not an insult,

---

1   (Granat, P.; "The demise of the independent doctor: a self-fulfilling prophecy?" *Journal of the Florida Medical Association*; 1988; Feb; 75(2): 105-7).

to call our "system" a "non-system." What about families, themselves? Are they "non-systems"? Yes, they are free to be who they want to be. Any "system" is safest in the hands of each patient and doctor, so that individual identity can have influence in such a personal relationship as that between doctor and patient. That is why plans to allow individuals control over their own money (vouchers from employers, with tax advantage) or the principle of medical savings accounts with catastrophic coverage, will restore choice and equity, with tax credits for individuals (most of us), and clinics for the needy. The truest "market" will prevail and "quality" will out, without millionaire (paid with our money) middle-persons and brokers that have characterized the HMO/government make-overs of medicine. Patients will come to us because we give them what they need, and they will pay for it.

Many of us have tried to practice, day to day, in a societally conscious, yet individually patient-conscious way, eschewing temptations to maximize our own earnings when unwarranted. (Example: coding conservatively consistent with effort expended). An entire coding industry has emerged, enriching only the code-changers, computer companies and book publishers. We are wound around rules.

Conversely, there are those of us who will game any system for maximum yields, aided by businesses, bureaucrats, and insurance and drug companies.

We have to wonder why people like Paul Ellwood and David Eddy are so often quoted as gurus, when it was they who promulgated the HMO route in the first place, leading clinicians to become administrators, trying to herd the rest of us like sheep (but we're cats, and you can't herd cats!). We have to wonder why people like Donald Berwick, MD, are given such credence, when he runs a huge impersonal "health" system, and has himself complained that his own desperately ill wife got lost in a huge morass, which could never have happened had she had a family doctor's name on her bracelet while in the hospital.

I particularly object to the so-called, population-based care "ideal," that cites failed systems such as Britain's and Canada's, and that rely on politically-correct estimations of which evidence constitutes the hallowed "evidence-base," when today's clinical "facts" are tomorrow's fictions in the blink of a mouse-click, or the latest soundbite. We all support research and useful population-based guidelines, when they fit our individual patient. We should be self-critical, if we are not accomplishing screening and preventive measure, so a certain amount of bean counting is acceptable. Certainly standards must be kept high, and accountability upheld. And I call now, as I called then in 1988 for more, not less, public-health expenditure and advertising toward targeted populations who are inattentive to healthy habits, to teach health-conscious attitudes and behaviors. The evidence is that habit change, more than wealth or medical care, is the more direct route to the good health of a population. Mass media can do more than physicians to change fads, fashions and behaviors.

Nevertheless, we are physicians, with in-depth and in-breadth training and not allied health professionals. Each special patient wants and needs our attention. The "population" can wait outside the examining room door. Many others can deliver "health care." Only we can reliably deliver medical care, complete with verifiable diagnoses, viable management over time, and most importantly, medical wisdom. The essence of care is a clinician's grasp of the accumulated evidence and guidelines applied to the special problems of one patient, not a population-based cookbook of lists. I am encouraged that the AAFP is redefining our professional identity. In doing so, let us not break faith with our ideals and professional goals, the grand traditions of healing expected by doctor and patient. Let us not break faith with that medical student who wrote so disconsolately. Let us not break faith with the very soul and body of medicine.

Your article showing the increased acute and long-term costs of longevity underscores the fallacy of expecting health system cost savings from enhanced health maintenance and curative care. Writing in *Scientific American* in April, 1995, Kristin Leutwyler amply showed data to support the idea that—although enormously important to well-being and quality of life—preventive care does not save money. It costs. And keeping people alive longer also costs. As personal physicians who support preventive care, we can educate our patients to pay directly for their usual and preventive care, without siphoning and diluting their money through government or insurance plans. Medical savings accounts would facilitate and enable them.

If patients believe their health is as worthwhile as a foreign vacation or new living room furniture, they will do so willingly. If they buy major medical insurance for accidents and illness, their risk will be spread. Medical indigents will need support for minimal basic care from the state, since no one should be denied basic care, but most people can budget for more in-depth needs which they deem worthy. We must be more honest with people and impart the news that staying alive must be part of their budget plan, like rent or food, in which the newly-identified need for long-term care will play an important part.

Sincerely,

Pepi Granat, M.D.

May, 2000

CHAPTER THIRTY-FOUR

Medicine on the Mend: A Fair and Final Fix

Never Before Proposed by Anyone in Defense of
Freedom and Autonomy for Doctors and Patients

Today a man came to my office. I asked, "Who referred you?" He said, "Actually, a magazine, *Miami Metro*." I had been lucky enough to have been listed in our areas "Best Doctors, as Rated by Their Peers." He was upset about his and his wife's prior care and was looking for a thorough exam and evaluation, and some answers to questions.

I mention this because—were there to be published a list of hospitals and physicians who adhere voluntarily to certain principles—the public (and the media) would take notice and benefit would accrue to those listed.

What principles? And what would motivate physicians and hospitals to participate?

Unless we look into the future, we're blind people, describing an elephant differently, depending on if we're holding the tail or the trunk. There are competing forces trying to shape "health care reform" while present forces push physicians into despair and patients out of the hospitals, sick and frustrated. Everyone sees it and all feel powerless. Yet there is real excellence and progress happening, and some physicians and companies are getting very rich—not necessarily in proportion to their excellence.

Certain facts are not disputed, regarding the condition of medical/health care today in this country. The first to go was freedom and autonomy, for both patients and physicians. They are captured and controlled by commercial entities, who are motivated by bottom lines, while mounting public relations campaigns saying they are for "quality." From commercial advocates (managed care) to social welfare advocates (cradle to grave government care), there appears to be no in-between offering, such as the fee-for-service concept, which is the most natural way people relate to each other. Yes, there were prior excesses, although they were few in number, but they gave that "system" a bad name. At least with fee-for-service, autonomy of patient and doctor was paramount. The patients forget that companies have only the money they (the patients, through their employers) give them. There are grains of truth in all the opposing forces, each accusing the other of not providing proper, equitable care. Most glaringly, there is nothing original coming from the doctors themselves—ourselves.

I would like to propose an entirely new idea—one which I've been advocating low-key in various venues, but as the deterioration of our beloved profession proceeds, and our grasp of control (for the good of the patients and the profession) is slipping badly, I feel compelled to speak more loudly. I believe this could work, but only if peas and pods of patients and the profession grab hold of it and run with it, seeing the equity and long-term reasonableness of it—with, above all, maintenance of freedom and autonomy for doctor and patient.

The proposal had three parts when first proposed in 2008: doctors, hospitals, insurance. Now, eleven years later, with drug prices through the roof, it needs four parts: doctors, drugs, hospitals, insurance. It could start without any new laws—by reasonable physicians and others seeing the rightness of it, and having the will to implement it.

The mission is to acknowledge and correct for the sins of commission and omission of both commerce (greed and mediocrity) and government (bureaucracy and mediocrity), to maintain freedom and autonomy, with incentives and rewards for effort and talent, but also for frugality and respect for resources, yet with ability to attract excellence because of sufficient (not excessive) promise of reward.

Jean-Jacques Rousseau spoke of the "social contract," by which reasonable people understood that mutual self-interest leads to behavior that enhances the benefits for each.[1]

---

[1]   The Social Contract, originally published as On the Social Contract; or, Principles of Political Right (French: *Du contrat social; ou Principes du droit politique*) by

The Doctors: The Ceiling Society

The Hospitals: The Manifesto

The Insurance: Medical Savings Accounts/Catastrophic Coverage

A patient looks in the *Miami Metro* magazine: he sees that Doctor X belongs to the Ceiling Society. He knows that these are the doctors who have agreed upon a "social contract" which will ultimately maintain excellence for the professions. He sees that Hospital Y has restructured itself along the same lines, and whether profit or non-profit, the executives are not empire-building and are adhering to the same principles as the doctors. And he sees insurance company Z, who provides a reasonable product for him to buy which spreads the risk, enabling catastrophic coverage.

The media's part is to devise clever ads that impart the message of spreading risk and what that means—encouraging young, healthy patients to insure themselves so as to assure the pool.

He votes with his feet—he goes to those doctors, insists on those hospitals, buys that insurance, and willing pays out of pocket for routine care (the gas and oil for his car).

Can this happen? Of course it can. It's a bandwagon thing—and the doctors and hospitals that begin will have been in the forefront. Just as the gentleman who came to my office today found me in *Miami Metro* magazine, so you will be listed. Consider the alternative: more of the present chaos, or a "universal" imposed system with all its bureaucracy. This idea is much different, and maintains the traditional American individuality and enterprise, along with elements of community spirit. It's a movement that's fair and that makes sense. Once it catches on it will become dominant, and will improve everyone's lives, giving more, not less, freedom. Perhaps it would take a grant from an interested philanthropy or think-tank. Or perhaps, we can do it just by our own will and imagination. But first, we

Jean-Jacques Rousseau, is a 1762 book in which Rousseau theorized about the best way to establish a political community in the face of the problems of commercial society, which he had already identified in his Discourse on Inequality (1755). [Retrieved from Wikipedia, April, 2021. See: https://en.wikipedia.org/wiki/The_Social_Contract.

must understand it and see the rightness and timeliness of it. Then it will happen. Shall we get started?

The Doctors: The Ceiling Society:

Objective: Eye on the Goal

The noble professions, to maintain their esteemed status, which is the real source of their value (both social and monetary), must rise above the fray, or risk ultimate devaluation. Pearl Buck, in her novel of revolutionary China, *The Good Earth*, often said of the uprisings that it always happens when "the rich get too rich." Those who may think this proposal may undermine, rather than strengthen, present status and earning ability, should think again. If "perception is reality" (even though we in medicine are definitely not all rich!) the general public will have "had enough" one day, and the professions will be thrown into chaos and servitude. Good generalists will be replaced with paraprofessionals, and specialists will not number a critical mass needed for progress and effectiveness. Medicine will enter a new dark age.

The fragile thread of that social contract is ours to weave wisely. Identifying with managed care and hospital survival, where bottom-line mentality rules will never advance our cause. The patient must always come first, not in hype, but in reality.

Background:

Physicians would wish to be paid for the work they do as physicians. If their talents command higher respect and value, or if they work long hours, they should be paid more, commensurately. Enterprise would be rewarded in a fee-for-service system, but up to a reasonable point. It is impossible to work more than twenty-four hours in a day. The earnings would stop at a properly high figure, perhaps the salary of the President of the United States.

Excesses over a given level of individual earnings would be either returned to patients or established in a backup fund for indigents, and/or research and teaching. There are social benefits to this, but also concerns. Is it anti-competitive? Members are free to belong or not and freely choose not to receive moneys not earned fairly. This would obviate the need for most regulations aimed at fraud and abuse.

Some might think that high earners and those of excellence would not have the "need" to join, and so could do well staying outside. And low earners have no need to join since they have no hope of "achieving" even the ceiling. But true excellence should include being able to see what real trouble all the professions are in with regard to their independence, autonomy and credibility. Countless regulations hamstringing professionals have their origins in excesses by the few who abuse their opportunities. And those of real excellence should be ready and willing to make a commitment to the "high road." Technical proficiency cannot substitute for professionalism.

Professional "competition" is not similar to business competition. We all want to give people "what they want," but often advertising and hype creates artificial wants while neglecting bona fide needs. This can become inappropriate at a professional level. The professions, themselves, with learning, licensing and appropriate regulatory procedures, have assured the public of at least minimum excellence of "product," where professions are concerned, though the marketplace may play some role, as perceptive people seek out superior, personal care.

Great wealth, because of its tendency to corrupt, should not be possible from professional activity. Now, with the advent of managed care, we must add that great wealth from business activity, involved with healing the sick, should not be possible. Why? Because managed organizations cannot practice medicine (or law, or engineering, etc.). Professions are different from business: they are the active fruition of a society's learning and wisdom. Their obligations derive from the good of the recipient, not the giver. Their principles are lasting and should not depend upon a fickle self-interested marketplace. The goals of a profession are unique. (This does not mean they should not be responsive to the public, borrowing the best concepts of good business; quite the opposite.)

Professionals are imparting knowledge and advice, and performing personal services, selling neither widgets, nor someone else's labor. There are only so many hours available, and it is the same twenty-four-hour day for all. Economies of scale for supplies, etc., go only a little way in minimizing expenses. It is not possible for there to be huge differences in income among physicians unless there is also some abuse of advantage. Talents and training are not that different (they *are* different, but not *that* different).

There is no way to increase production very much except by overpricing, or some other gimmick. By the same reasoning, with managed care, there is no way to decrease cost without eventually decreasing services, especially when the dollar pays mainly for executives and profit, not medical care.

Examples

In law, the acceptance of unconscionable contingency fees and/or "referral fees," or tainted drug-dealer moneys.

In medicine, the windfall of maintaining the high price of a new, originally-expensive and infrequently-performed procedure when it becomes less expensive and many can be done in a day, such as arthroscopies, gastroscopies.

In both fields, the scandalous handling and padding of workers compensation cases to their own advantage, with no attempt to arrive at the truth nor to save the taxpayers one cent).

The entire RBRVS (Resource-Based Relative Value Scale) costing millions to research, implement and administer, was based upon the assumptions of fairly apportioned time and talent, in an attempt to equalize the earning field, which had become crazily skewed. When the few high-priced procedural physicians ceased being the recipients of unconscionable earnings, they became the victims, due to managed care's capture and control of doctors and patients. Now, the unconscionable profits have shifted to executives and managers.

How To Get To Goal

Establish the principles that:

1. We do not want to be paid for what we don't do for patients (capitation)

2. We will treat patients based on their needs alone, within prudent cost and best practices guidelines, since ultimately, all moneys come from patients

3. We will belong voluntarily to the Ceiling Society: if our earnings from practicing medicine exceed $250,000 (or whatever number is decided upon, net, after expenses; investment and other income not included) we will redistribute the overage either among all patients who have paid us, or into a fund for the needy. We will sign no contracts except with patients. Our "business" is first and always with the patient.

4. We will fund the distribution of a directory in which are listed all physicians agreeing to these principles. This will be our only expense for this "mending of medicine"

5. We will advocate excellent public health announcements, an investment long overdue by our federal and state governments

6. We will advocate Medical Savings Accounts, so that people can keep their own money and pay us directly, instead of well people sending money to insurance plans

7. We will advocate reasonable catastrophic insurance for all to spread true risk.

8. We will volunteer for clinics for the needy, and encourage state and county governments to establish them for those falling through the cracks.

9. We will encourage individual responsibility, not corporate handholding among our patients.

10. We will realize that freedom for doctor and patient is a positive value. Today's trends are not "here to stay" necessarily, but may collapse of their own weight and poor principles, leaving one doctor caring for one patient in the ancient contract of faith in each other.

The Hospitals: The Manifesto

The Issue

A hospital remains the place where physicians, the only ones who can practice medicine, can take their patients for in-patient care when office care will not suffice.

That is all a hospital is and should be. Attempting to "vertically integrate" care means taking over a piece of each patient-doctor encounter which occurs *outside* the hospital, bringing it into the hospital, and culling a piece of the financial action of that encounter as well. This is unnecessary, spreads the patients' resources to those who are not caring for them, is costly to the patient and the system, and eventually counterproductive for patient care.

There are plenty of dollars out there for patient care: they're being distributed to everyone but doctors and nurses. Of all aggregated medical costs, physicians get $0.19 to $0.21 cents of each dollar, of which over half is overhead. This means $0.10 for us. With current changes, it will be even *less*.

The attempt of hospitals to become something besides a place for a physician to take his/her sick patient is not relevant to patient care, but is very relevant to other interests.

There are those who would have us believe that "survival" of a hospital depends on entering into unsound practices, such as control of medical care being wrested out of the hands of physicians, and into the hands of administrators, insurance plans and insurance companies.

The fact that this is going on all over the country does not make it right.

"Alignment of incentives" and "assuming risk" are merely phrases used by organizations and hospitals who are only interested in medicine as a vehicle to make money. Physicians assumed maximal risk just by going into Medicine, and continue to assume risk by hanging out their shingles. Although physicians assumed they would earn a living by *doing* medicine, they went into it for the purpose of practicing *medicine*. As soon as they *stop* doing that, they become business-persons, and the proper aim becomes achieving dollars.

There is one way to "align incentives." That is to optimize conditions for the true aims of the practice of medicine (getting and keeping people well), paying all physicians a reasonable amount based on real work done, and plowing any excess profits back into patient care, and using hospitals to get the job done only when absolutely needed.

Physicians should earn money based on the practice of medicine only (apart from outside investments), and should charge a reasonable fee based on work done. They should be free to set those fees wherever they wish, within existing law. No one, physicians or other persons, should profit personally from any hospital enterprise. Any other businesses connected with medicine, lab, x-ray, food service, etc., that could be seen to make a "profit" for the hospital, would expect to plow those profits right back into the hospital and would not accrue to any persons delivering care. (Of course, any services should receive fair value, but only for those services actually performed and needed). In fact, physicians connected with the hospital could be encouraged to contribute to a research and education fund. A more unusual (though standard at universities) method might be for physicians (voluntarily) to decide to earn only up to a ceiling (which would be quite high, but not exorbitant) and would return anything over that into such a fund to be run by the Foundation. That would solve the problem that the Relative Value Scale couldn't fix and would make this hospital enormously popular with patients. They would know that *no one* was abusing the system, and all their dollars would come back around to them, either in the form of actual care or as investment in the means to give them care in the future. Physicians would act on what they know now: that the skills of any one of us are not so greatly different as our incomes.

- The hospital will declare itself self-pay only. No insurance will be accepted directly. When insurance companies (and even Medicare) see how little it actually costs here, compared to what others are paying, they'll be beating down the doors to reimburse the patients who come here.

- Real and actual costs will be charged to patients. There will be absolutely *no* cost-shifting. An aspirin will cost what an aspirin costs. The administration of that aspirin will be charged as such, and the actual cost will be calculated and charged.

- All nurses will be private contractors, preferably organized in pods which operate floor by floor, working in the same place whenever possible. They will provide for the total nursing care in their units. There will be some measure of physician staff input into nursing decisions, instead of complete autonomy on the part of the nursing staff.

- All lab work will be contracted out unless it can be proven to be done cheaper in house (not the other way around). The present lab will be a stat lab only. The stat services of other labs, if faster and cheaper, will also be contracted out. Whenever any lab fails to perform, the contract will be switched to one who will fulfill the high standards of the hospital.

- All radiology will be contracted out. The present equipment will be bought out by whomever can offer the best bid. The radiology coverage must include stat coverage.

- The OR will be under the medical staff. It will function as it presently does, but with privately contracted nurses as well. Pods of nurses can band together to offer services.

- All food service will be contracted out, unless proof of cheaper in-house service. There will be the opportunity for four classes of luxury in food service, basic, nice, fine, deluxe. (Of course the diets prescribed will have to be honored as well).

- Cleaning and housekeping will be contracted out, unless proof of cheaper in-house service.

- No capital "improvement" will occur without debate and approval of the entire medical staff.

- All administrative functions will not consume more than ten (10%) percent of the entire budget.

- The room fee will be just that—a room fee. The operation of the housing at the hospital could be also contracted out to a hotel company. Nothing but the actual cost of the room will be included. There will be four types of rooms and service. Nursing service which is essential will be separated from attendant service which is merely desirable and a luxury: Basic—ward service, four in a room, no phone, no TV, common bathroom.: Nice—one step up; Fine— another step up; Deluxe—super-duper. These can be refined by the "hotel" mentality and management.

- Modern methods of energy conservation, including solar heating, will be utilized in every way possible.

- Recycling and reusing will be instituted. No disposables will be used unless absolutely necessary for infectious purposes.

- There will be no "marketing" or advertising other than word of mouth and discreet placement of tasteful articles in newspapers and journals. Physicians will participate in informational programs if desired to get the word out.

- Equity participation by users of the hospital. The cornerstone of this project will be to provide the very best care at half the cost to patients willing to pay up front for it. They can work out payment plans, special arrangements with banks, or use credit cards as a last resort. For every dollar a patient spends at the hospital, he/she will get a portion back in the form of health credits to be applied to his/her own future medical bills, or those of a designate. Thereby, loyalty to the hospital will be achieved, and an incentive to spend discretionary dollars here rather than elsewhere. The exact formula, year by year, will depend upon how frugal the hospital was the year before, thereby keeping costs down. Employees and medical staff will receive a slightly higher "rebate" for using the hospital services.

- No travel expenses will be paid for administrative staff unless absolutely essential to the day-to-day running of the hospital.

- The business of taking care of patients and keeping up with developments in Medicine will be the only business activities of this hospital. No ancillary attempts to make money will be needed, since the patients will pay for what they get, and there will be no frills for the basic package. The frills which may be elected will be designed to make a modest profit to assure excess budget for indigent care. Raising money (Mercury Ball, etc.) to supplement indigent care or worthy hospital projects would be encouraged.

- Ten percent of the budget will go to indigent care, from the earnings of the hospital. When that 10% is reached, no more indigent care will be possible. The county will have to receive those patients, or work out a subsidy. Of course, our responsibility to render emergency care (true emergency, not clinic care) remains, but that could be worked out.

- Meetings involving paid personnel will be kept to a bare minimum to satisfy any regulatory requirements only.

- Paperwork and mailings will be kept to a bare minimum, using boxes where doctors can pick up notices instead of multiple mailings. Use of fax when costs are thereby lowered will be encouraged.

- Education and library information systems will be given due attention and should not be cut unless necessary, but information systems and their support should be analyzed carefully for the best buys. All support from donors and companies should be accepted as long as no strings are attached, and all arrangements are up-front.

- Chief of Nursing will set standards and manage the privately-contracted nursing pods. The only employees of the hospital will be one layer of administration, their secretaries and support staff. They will coordinate all activities not in the nursing sphere.

- The board of governors will be a working board, informing and receiving input from the medical staff. It will decide the direction of the hospital, but will not present the medical staff with plans for which there is no possibility of control or change, once made.

- The income of the doctors on staff will be from the practice of medicine within their own offices, or from agreed-upon contracted *medical* services which they, themselves perform. No other "business" opportunities shall be presented to them or others by which to profit from the operations of this hospital.

+ No conflict of interest between board members and opportunities at the hospital should be permitted.

+ The hospital will price its services so as to afford necessary updates of equipment to stay on the forefront of medical advances.

+ The hospital, as an entity will divest itself from the practice of medicine in any form. There will be no salaried physicians at this hospital, unless to augment earnings to assure a minimum floor of earnings for a necessary service. Reason: the aim of the hospital changes from a place for an independent doctor to bring an independent patient to be taken care of, to a place which is maximizing its earning capacity on its own, with the doctor very subservient to the economic health of the hospital. It is an unhealthy incestuous arrangement. Contracts for necessary services which must be ongoing, such as radiology and pathology will be allowed and must conform to the needs of the hospital. If long-term contracts are necessary for security of both parties, that would be allowed.

+ Any office space will be rented at fair market value; any services provided will also be at market value.

Fulfilling The Circle—
Life and Death Issues: Motivation, School,
Sport, Weather, Environment, Choices,
Literature, Food, History, Peace, Forensics,
Aging, Dying, Music

CHAPTER THIRTY-FIVE

Spiritual Chemistry

I was standing on my head in the lotus position when it came to me: what I was here for, what I was supposed to do in the world, and how it would all end.

My friend and I had decided that our organic chemistry course would sink in better with more blood to our brains. At least that's what the yoga books had said. So we faced each other, concentrating on equations, our heads nestled in palms interlaced, our elbows forming the base triangle, our legs in the air, neatly folded, ankles pinned under thighs, knees out tailor-like, our backs perfectly straight.

I had shopped for religion years before, going to a different church or synagogue each Sunday, coming away with a profound and calming sense of reverence—induced mostly by the music and art of it all—and an envy of those who were able to believe.

But the confusion and clash with logic and history blocked my acceptance of any of the tenets, and the plethora of beliefs reassured me that no one of them could be held closely. I was at the scattered time of life, when nothing makes much sense, when you're figuring out who you are and where you're going.

Though all of life is turning out to be like that, the early days are the worst, since you're just getting used to living in your own changing body.

I had planned to be an English teacher, inspired by great teachers right here in Miami-Dade County. But I had switched to science halfway through college, having discovered the pure beauty of concrete thought, and having tired of the relativity of art. But I had no idea what I would do with my new affinity, since my natural tendencies were more humanistic.

One day, browsing in a bookstore, I came upon a book called *Concentration*, written by a yogi. It translated eastern philosophy and mind/body control into a useful method for westerners. I did the exercises, both mental and physical, leaving out the part about the ultimate aim of the game: becoming nothing at all, one with the universe. I figured I had lots of time for that.

Then it came, in a hot, late afternoon—standing on my head—just as the yogi had promised![1] Was it more blood to the brain? Was it the joy of my friend's smile, and our vulnerability, as we tested how long we could study on our heads? I was in the middle of reciting an equation, one we had forgotten but, suddenly, could remember, when the revelation broke through, and I knew: I would be a physician. I would use this organic chemistry; I would learn more—enough to help my fellow-creatures make it through this life when afflicted. I would find my special place. Suddenly I was sure what I was doing here. I also knew I would write about it.

---

[1]   An important disclaimer is in order here. It's actually not a good idea for anyone with arthritis, osteoporosis, any history of neck injury, anyone with hypertension (high blood pressure), aneurysms (usually unknown), or glaucoma to start standing on their head. In fact, it's probably not a good idea for healthy people either. And as for the claim that standing on one's head brings increased intelligence or learning, I'm sure this was a bit of wishful thinking, perhaps hoping to the attain Nirvana a bit more quickly.

CHAPTER THIRTY-SIX

Where Did You Train?

It's back to school for the kids. Can you remember it—wondering if you could start over, make new friends, forget last year's problems, turn over a new leaf?

The real beginning of the year, September.

But for many children and teenagers, back-to-school does not hold the promise it did for us. Many are being neither educated nor trained; neither literate nor fit for a job. They are in limbo because of lack of direction.

The Doctor Learns

From where does guidance come? On Wednesdays, when I leave the office, I'm enlightened by listening to the school board meeting on WLRN, National Public Radio, 91.3 FM. If your kids are in private school or out of school, it's still worthwhile, because our taxes are being used for everyone's kids, and our town is being robbed by those going astray.

Going sour starts somewhere—and today, that could mean not just neighborhoods, but schools. Why? Because it is the peer group that contributes greatly to raising kids today and school is where they meet. As nuclear and extended family life weakens, the school assumes more meaning and becomes the extended family of the child or teen. Even if home life is very strong, outside influences are too powerful for most to resist.

Teachers do heroic jobs but cannot do the impossible. Many believe throwing more money at the system would help; as in medicine, more money usually ends up in a top-heavy administrative, bureaucratic hierarchy instead of where it belongs: in the hands of the nitty gritty workers, the teachers themselves. What if we paid floor nurses much more than hospital administrators, and teachers more than superintendents?

Schools and school systems will be changing and the directions depend on everyone's input, in the neighborhoods and at the polls.

Medicine is accustomed to interfacing with school health, and volunteering in matters of health in the schools. Many of us physicians in the DCMA went into the schools in May for the AIDS "blitz" of education, lecturing and talking with the kids to enlighten them on the scourge of AIDS. Many of us take on unsung, individual projects. (We're interested to know of your own special input into any school: please write and tell us about it.)

We have precious opportunities to influence and direct children. The same tale told by a parent has a whole new meaning when reaffirmed by a physician. We tend to underestimate how our words ring in people's ears—and especially in children's.

The Doctor Counsels

Almost all specialties include children and teens. Because their health is generally good, it's likely that regular contact with a pediatrician or family doctor (apart from immunizations) will not be more frequent than being seen for broken bones, rashes, allergies, tonsils or other specialty-oriented problems.

Along with competent care by subspecialists it helps when kids get some attention to developmental and social problems. A bit of encouragement, a pat on the back to reinforce acceptable behaviors, a caring contact that says to them, "You're okay; I have confidence in you" goes a long way, especially from a physician. A smidgen of interest in their extracurricular activities, as well as a question as to how they're doing in school and whether there are any problems, can help direct them to other specialists (not necessarily medical), or back to their pediatrician or family doctor to solve the problem behind the obvious one presented.

The Doctor Guides

Although the goal always is to produce self-direction, children and teens cannot be left alone in a sea of clamoring distractions. They need guidance and feedback.

We can find out if family members are able to guide the child or if help is needed from social agencies. Much is written now about child abuse; looking at the larger problem of failure to maximize children's potential would widen the lens of scrutiny to encompass and find solutions not only to abuse, but to other ills.

The Doctor Influences

School policies can be influenced by the physician-citizen. If we believe that education is different from training, and that some persons are simply more suited for one or the other, then that point of view could be made known. It does not benefit a child to attempt to educate him/her beyond her/his desires or capabilities, nor should anyone aspiring to extra studies be denied the opportunity.

Other ideas may surface. I have thought, for example, that each family with children should have longitudinal contact with either a counselor or an assigned teacher or even a trained volunteer, throughout the school years, from entry to exit of the school system. Progress and milestones of each child and family can be followed; there will be someone out there who cares. An advocate within the system could help and be immediately available. Early intervention for solving problems will be more fruitful. This occurs now unofficially, whenever a teacher takes a special interest in child and his/her family; it could become a permanent and ongoing project. It could interface with state agencies when needed, to yield cost-effective results. The new "Mentors Program," connected to the "Cities in Schools" effort, is exactly a right step in that direction. Cross-sectional, episodic, disconnected attempts at intervention would seem less effective.

The Doctor Cares

Will there be guidance for children and teens? As we return to the season of learning, which is never out of style, how can we season the sauce for the kids? How can we help each to amplify the natural, best path toward a happy niche in the mesh of society's web? What combination of training and education will serve them best? What was it for us? Can we reach back and recall? Did we receive more direction than we remember, and are we caring to help pass it on?

CHAPTER THIRTY-SEVEN

Gee—You're a Real Sport

Sport and medicine cross paths often. Apart from injuries sustained by sportsmen and women, the way equilibrium of mind and body must be maintained in training and performance, brings sports and medicine into commonality of purpose and method. Both can keep us together, or tear us apart.

The feeling of teamwork, of clicking toward a common goal, is one of nature's finest highs, attainable in team sports, in the operating room, and in the well-run office on a good day. The sense of limitless power in well-trained muscles, doing the brain's every command, every nuance—responding under pressure to relentless challenge is experienced alike by marathoners and interns, after a night on call. The discipline, practice, concentration and attention to detail required in both sports and medicine, the concept of keeping one's eye on the ball, of aiming high and fulfilling goals, both of one's own or others, are all found in medicine and in sports.

Physicians are fascinated by others who achieve, though in a different field. That doctors may even compete, switch careers or become creditable amateurs is not surprising. That they may attempt to enter the rarefied atmosphere of fame and fortune accorded the modern-day heroes of sports by serving as their physicians and mentors is helpful for the health and future of those who entertain the rest of us with their extraordinary exploits on the fields, rings and courts of the world.

Fun and games go together—or do they? Are we having fun yet? A question implying we should be, but maybe aren't. Sports can also be no fun at all. A recent example of misplaced objectives is the baseball strike—fun for no one.

It would seem that sport leads to an enhanced confidence. Possibly that's true for fewer persons than we think. In sports, one person's glory can be another's humiliation. The toddler learns the difference between his own toy and his playmate's. One of the first instincts is, "Mine!" Soon, in playful tussles, it's the victory which becomes his. Then, at school in "free play," informal competition establishes ascendancy, usually dependent on size within groups of the same age. Then the teams are chosen. In those early years, size largely determines apparent sports ability. The small child is chosen last; even if he can throw or kick well, he can't throw or kick far. Occasionally, wit and coordination can make up for size, while two left feet, or obesity, or hand-eye deficits can negate its advantage.

Unlike math or language, where ability-grouping prevents embarrassment faced by a slow-learner in a normal class, physical education classes do not usually classify by ability or by size. For all but the stars, both learning and self-esteem may suffer. The chances to build life-long exercise skills and to associate vigorous physical activity with pleasurable and socially-reinforcing emotions are lost. Kids can be traumatized by these early public humiliations. Kids are honest; they won't pick a runt just to be nice. They'll always pick him/her last—for every team. Being always picked last in front of everyone sends the obvious message, "nobody wants me." True, it may spur such children on to greater heights in other fields, since they fail so dismally in sports: some of them even become doctors.

In the special world of professional sports, only boxing and wrestling, despite other drawbacks, understand that size counts. What if we had basketball teams not restricted only to the tallest (because of obvious advantage with a fixed basket height) but grouped by height, as fighters are grouped by weight? The baskets could be adjusted up or down with a fixed ratio to the height range of the players. Why are the laws of physics, biology and sociology not used more in consonance with human realities by physicians, physical educators, the school systems and the sports systems? The shorter, lighter men and women might even give us a faster, more exciting run for our money. Certainly, equal talents in basketball populate all height groups. Why are only the tallest afforded a chance to reach the top? One could look at other sports as well, to truly "level the playing field," consistent with human possibilities.

Sports and games have long done duty as metaphor for life, for strife, for drama, for fairness, for justice, for change, for chance, for war, for peace and for health and healing.

In competition there is glory; there can be heroes and villains. In conflict there is resolution. Sport is an outlet for pent-up energy, especially in young men. It is a chance to fight in an acceptable milieu. High levels of male hormone build muscle mass and aggressive characteristics, and are physiologic in teens and early twenties. Male animals traditionally must spar, usually for territory or reproductive advantage. Sports are better and safer than war, and get more attention than a dating service.

The intense, hypnotic draw of sports stars and teams to lure masses, spending fortunes on tickets and wagers, and even losing lives in stampedes, attests to the power of sports to capture the imagination of individuals and entire nations.

Like a good story, or a case in medicine, each contest brings anticipation, a beginning, middle, suspense, a climax and then the end. There is an aftermath and later, memories. That's fun. The satisfying part stems from the tension/resolution inherent in every game: a finite, manageable entity having a suspenseful, unknown end. Then it's over until next time.

As in medicine the outcome has too many variables to make sure prediction possible. Sports and medicine are both games in which—all else being nearly equal—chance may play a vital role. The secret thought that it could have been different, that it could have gone either way, makes it possible for all losers to be not just "also-rans" but imaginary winners.

Being "a real sport," means understanding, with equanimity, the pitfalls of being human, and how reality often fails to meet expectation, lessons learned incessantly, over and over again, in both sport and medicine.

CHAPTER THIRTY-EIGHT

Andrew, How Could You?

"From the road I saw the exposed inside of one kitchen, naked in the sunshine, pouring down where the roof had been, the doors ripped off the china cabinet, the teacups still hanging by their stems."

Everyone has his/her own "war story" of Hurricane Andrew. Here's mine.

I had volunteered for the disaster committee at South Miami Hospital. During the storm, we saw shattered windows, patients moved to hallways, other doctors' in-patients "crashing" and needing urgent attention, pregnant women and families filling corridors, and an amazing smoothness of operation by the administration, with minimal disruption even of complicated services. For example, a patient developed copious rectal bleeding and we were able to get ICU (Intensive Care Unit) support, blood, (Lynn Leverett, MD), a gastroenterology consult (Dr. Lawrence Rothman) a nuclear bleeding scan (Dr. Robert Gordon), and take her to surgery (Dr. George Brener), all during the storm and just after.

Many others, unsung and unnamed (you know who you are) deserve plaudits. I was proud of "my hospital," especially its nurses, and our medical staff president, Dr. Joseph Traina, who was responsible for the smooth working of the medical staff and the disaster committee.

My daughter, a University of Miami medical student, and four friends stayed at our house in Coral Gables, built in 1937. On Monday, the day of the storm, I ventured home, only six miles. It was like driving in uncharted woods. I, a native Miamian, hardly knew where I was! Landmarks were gone. Streets were covered with fallen trees, lines and street signs were down, usual routes of access were blocked. I found most of the beautiful banyans of Bird Road uprooted in the south lane. I wound around downed trees with the car, hoping not to get stuck in the mud. I found my house, solid as a rock; the yard was almost a loss, with favorite trees broken and downed, the fence broken. We had missed the eye, and a good house holds.

I returned to camp out at the hospital for two more days, and was witness to so many people doing heroic duty. There were our own nurses plus volunteer nurses from Melbourne and other places up-state, and from South Carolina, who were "paying us back" for our own kindness during Hugo. It was a time to be proud of the human race. (Until three days later when price gougers attempted to extract $500 for a simple electrical job that cost $150!)

Then, I was able to get to our farm in the Redland, a lime and avocado grove in its prime, personally planted and nurtured for twelve years as a family project and hope for the future, but I was unprepared for what I saw!

The entire lime grove was…*gone!* The trees were not even there—blown away. The avocado grove was like scrambled spaghetti, no leaf nor fruit on any tree. Every tree either cracked, split or uprooted, some completely dead and out of the ground. But at least the avocado trees were *there*. The lime trees were not; it looked like before we ever planted. There had been big, fruitful, beautiful trees—one thousand of them.

A house can be rebuilt in six months. Lime trees take three years even to grow—six to be productive. Avocados longer. Our Redland neighbor told us the eye had passed over; he had come out to stillness and stars, then a freight train roaring. There were things I'd always wanted to do that I got to do: climbing from limb to limb and tree to tree, in the tops of twenty-foot-high trees, like a squirrel except that the trees were lying on their sides, toppled in both directions, their tops kissing. And I was climbing because there was no other way to get around them.

Our neighbor's house was fine, but others were devastated. From the road, I saw the exposed inside of one kitchen, naked in the sunshine pouring down where the roof had been, the doors ripped off the china cabinet, the teacups still hanging by their stems. I could only think of all the private histories, the baby pictures. We share common stories and common guilt: we know we should not mourn for ourselves when so many others are worse off.

But our own hurts are ours; we have learned to nurse them, carefully pick ourselves up, brush the debris from our streets and our minds, reach out and help when we can, and move along.

Life is like a hurricane: it has a calm eye. Then it hits you again when you think you're all right.

CHAPTER THIRTY-NINE

Connections and Consolations

Years ago, when I told my immigrant grandmother that I wanted to go into medicine, she took me by the shoulders and looked into my eyes.

"Why do you want to be around sickness and death?" she said. "Do something where you can laugh and be happy."

For a minute it made sense then, almost without thinking, I blurted out, "But the sickness and death will be there, even if I'm not around to see it. Knowing it's there, and that I'm not doing anything about it, doesn't let me laugh and be happy, either."

She thought about that—and never tried to dissuade me again.

Last mid-winter, I took an old friend, an oncologist from the frigid northeast, to Fairchild Tropical Gardens, a special place, dear to me, where my friends and I used to study as University of Miami students in the 1950s. She felt the peace and power of the spellbinding tropical gardens, a place to "behold the evident processes of nature and be consoled by them."[1]

In medicine, we too have the experience of witnessing the incredible power of healing, and pure aesthetic beauty such as the acid-base juggling act of the kidney. But how much more often do we, as physicians, behold the evident processes of nature and are appalled by them? How ugly is the putrescence and tumescence we see in our patients with infections and cancer? We become used to it: it doesn't offend or scare us any more. Yet, we must maintain our own consolation in the face of the misery and despair around us, our daily diet. One human life at a time constitutes our field of work, and the old move over for the young.

---

1 Dr. Liberty Hyde Bailey, biologist, in his dedication speech, delivered in 1938.

But what about earth? There can be no replacement. Remedies are being prescribed to cure the planet's ills. We must each become newly aware of creative, cooperative solutions to earth's many problems. I didn't know, when my grandmother confronted me, that although we may "cure seldom, alleviate often and comfort always," there will also be helplessness in the face of forces that can't be affected. We can now do a lot, but still never enough for our own patients. That is when we can retreat to gardens and wilderness (but only if we act to preserve them), whether in the spring or winter of our lives, fix our gaze upon the cycle of life in other organisms, and reflect upon our place in the ongoing, renewing chain. Note: this was written in anticipation of the "Earth Summit" conference in Rio de Janeiro, Brazil, June, 1992. On August 24, 1992, Hurricane Andrew profoundly changed and nearly destroyed the gardens, but scientists from around the world have convened to save its rare plants and palms. We will have the Fairchild Tropical Gardens back.

CHAPTER FORTY

The Physician's Role in Environmental Awareness

Physician, Heal Thy Earth

As physicians, the health of each patient is our chief sphere, yet the global condition of our planet concerns us. Our collective consciousness can set an improved reality into orbit. What can we use in our daily decisions—not just in medicine (our own offices and hospitals) but in our private lives—that makes a difference where "saving the planet' is concerned?

Perhaps we should just leave it up to "experts" to set the pace, and hope to follow along in time. But maybe our pooled wisdom, scientifically and socially, is needed—and even wanted—in the effort to maximize our natural heritage.

We have some influence in our communities and hospitals, we talk to patients, we set examples, we have some overlapping expertise which applies. The articles presented in this issue are only a fraction of what can be said on the subject of both earth's preservation and the welfare of human beings, a concept called sustainable development. This may be a fertile field for an annual issue and update on the condition of Patient Earth, and our human condition. Who of us does not agonize over the drought and famine in Somalia right now, yet shrink in dismay to hear that food and supplies, generously sent and well-meant, are diverted by thugs and young, needy men, never reaching the neediest victims?

Without sufficient food supply, sending seeds to replant farms, even if there is rain, would likely be thwarted by starving individuals, eating the seeds before they are put into the ground!

Individually we will have little effect, if any. Together we can exert significant impact. Each of the authors has a contribution which fills in a piece of the puzzle, and a point of view with which you may agree or argue. We would be happy to stimulate both, and will welcome and publish any responsible counterpoint.

New data stream in, as they do in medicine, changing points of view and plans of action. Our own actions at home and at the polls are dependent upon our conclusions, which depend upon having more than a passing acquaintance with new concepts.

We can try to:

+ make sense of the varied agendas of political entities, environmental organizations, and calls for help and funds among sorely-strapped yet needy and worthwhile causes.

+ sift out fact from fiction, among the scientific and pseudoscientific claims behind advice and courses of action.

+ cast a jaundiced eye equally upon media, government and private reports when they are politically or meanly motivated, and attempt to sort out the truth—always impossible—yet worth a try.

+ seek out and change our own habitual ways of reacting, wasting, consuming, even thinking, if—after due consideration based on education and open-mindedness—we deem those ways counter-productive toward the goal of a healthy planet.

Although we can help each other to see things more distinctly—especially on a clear day—each one of us must do the lonely job of thinking and changing ourselves.

CHAPTER FORTY-ONE

My Father's Mango Tree

Lovingly, he would place the fish heads in the hole, dug just so deep, and would cover them gently with leaves and pieces of palm fronds. Then he would shovel the dirt back over them, leaving no remnant, so the cats wouldn't think to dig them back up. Satisfied, he would look up at the only daughter of his five who had any interest in his growing of roses, radishes, tomatoes and mangos, and who watched all that he did in the garden with fascination and wonder.

He would smile, and crinkle his eyes, his bald head shining in the sun. I would smile back, afraid to ask whether planting fish heads would grow new fish. He would pat me on the head, and give me a fat, wet kiss on my forehead. Later, when I found out why he planted fish heads, along with many other things about my father, I marveled at how kids take everything in stride, at face value, until they live long enough to gain perspective and do their own planting.

When I traveled in India I marveled at all the vegetation from home I recognized. These days, with out-sourcing to India, and an Indian voice on the phone when you need computer support, we might feel alienated. Not me. I have more in common with them than with my fellow Americans, who only know apples. At least they know about mangos. Here in Florida, even the north Floridians don't know about mangos, unless they see them in the market.

My father's mango tree bore such delicious fruit that neighbors and friends would clamor for them, even if they had their own tree. And when my parents sold their house in mid-Miami Beach to move to their dream of living on the water, they placed a codicil on the deed, so that they would have mango rights in perpetuity.

My father only had daughters. When I became pregnant (before ultrasound), two of my sisters had three daughters among them. After a trip back to Florida to take my Medical Boards, my father drove me to the airport and as I boarded the plane back to New Haven, I said good-bye to him, not knowing it would be for the last time, promising him that with this baby, he finally would have his boy. He died three months later on Valentine's day, four weeks before my son was born.

My mother outlived him by many years, and lives on, unseeing and unknowing, these last eight years. As her Alzheimer's disease progressed, one of the few things she relished was being fed mangos, dimly reviving inaccessible, sweet memory. My father's mango tree was a Haden. The mangos were so sweet, so delicious,; they seemed to have dropped from heaven, ambrosia, the fruit of the gods. Today, I ate someone's Haden mango from his tree. Oh, it was good—but nothing like my father's. Once, I tasted one just like his; I suspected there were fish heads.

CHAPTER FORTY-TWO

The Secret Ingredients

A recent, artful Mexican movie, "Like Water for Chocolate," reminds us how bound up our food is with the basic emotions and rhythms of life, how we relate our drives and memories to early tastes and smells which become the essences of the richness and fluidity of our substantial selves.

In medical practice, our task is often to assess and make changes in a fairly ordinary matter, our patients' choice of foods. Yet such a basic item as what patients eat from day to day, and their prior experience with food or perhaps eating disorders, may be unknown to us, unless we ask for details.

We may not know immediately what to do with the information, and many purveyors of dietary supplements and so-called diet advice are quick to say that physicians don't have formal "nutrition" training in medical school. In medical school we had quite a lot of nutrition information, but it was scattered in various courses. Structure of vitamins and their chemistry was covered in biochemistry, mechanisms in physiology, deficiency diseases in pathology, drug use in pharmacology, etc.

In junior year, we went to luncheons put on by the dietary department at Jackson, where we ate (on pain of failing the course) a different type of hospital meal each week, and were lectured on the indications for ordering each diet, etc. I remember the effect it had on us—just realizing that we would be in charge of something as personal as what someone must eat, day after day.

The low-fat diet then was dry and tasteless, requiring much water to moisten the food. I can still feel the cardboard quality of the food sticking to my mouth as I gulped water to wash it down. We joked about it then. Now it's serious.

The most important thing we learned was how to learn more. Researchers have begun to scratch the interface between nutrition and longevity, and freedom from various diseases. We know more about mechanisms: theories and hypotheses have a modicum of proof, evidence pours in daily, and the food industry has come up with more palatable ways of enduring restrictions.

The themes of this and the preceding two issues seem to form a natural trilogy: "The Swing of the Pendulum" (April), "Alternative Medicine" (May) and "Nutrition." All have wide range of opinion, folklore, fact, changing studies and confusing evidence, and the tendency of various sectors of the public and different specialties within medicine, to be clutching at different appendages of the elephant, like the proverbial six blind men.

A different creature indeed is perceived by each. It is no wonder that food habits are difficult to change. Even if all could agree on optimal nutrition, the art and beauty of food, the culture and presentation of food, the memories and fantasies of food, the wisdom and folly of food, are beyond mere science, beyond behavioral quick fixes. When we talk seriously about food, we trample into the bounds of love. To change ingrained symbols takes powerful persuasion. To nourish images of warm well being, somewhere in our diets must be—like the water, which achieves fine chocolate—the secret ingredients of hope and love.

CHAPTER FORTY-THREE

Telling and Retelling History:
Who Owns the Past?

It is fitting in this year of the 50th anniversary of the end of World War II, when many are contesting others' versions of the truths of that ignominious and heroic era, that we are looking at our own history and reflecting on its truths. January's issue, combined with March, joins many stories that we can savor, as we look at our place in the medical continuum.

Medicine has come through many historical hurdles. There have been forces for good and evil. We are now caught in a force which appears relentless, as did the events of the war, yet which could have been, and still could be, reversed by our will and action, if only we would see the future evils as our successors will, and rise up and throw them off.

Much of our present activity involves identifying with the aggressors. We are making Faustian pacts with devils, hoping to gain salvation, or at least comfort and security right now, until we retire or our kids go to college. But history moves in forever directions. We can't go back but we can regress.

What is so wrong with going with the flow? Letting history sweep us along? Then revising events to suit us, changing our history books when the truth is too painful?

When the signal events of the twentieth century are told, in addition to the debate about how to remember the Auschwitz death camp and the bombing of Hiroshima, there will need to be a footnote on the demolition of the freedoms of American patients and physicians and the selling to the lowest bidders of a noble (yet flawed) historically independent profession.

Mark Twain said that the very ink that history is written in is liquid prejudice. We choose to remember and retell that which is consonant with our deepest fears, or our most wishful thinking. Drs. Simpson, Brown and Waters retelling of the Black experience in Dade County, enlightens us and illuminates our own narrow views. We are reminded that we miss much of what is going on all around us.

We hear from some historians that it is the powerful and the dominant who get to control history. The facts rarely matter much; it is the lessons to be learned that seem to count, according to Gustav Niebuhr, writing in the *New York Times*, January 29, 1995.

In Poland, despite the correction by facts and Polish scholars themselves of the fallacy that half those killed were Poles, rather than ninety percent Jews, Poland draws an image of national martyrdom from the memory of the death camp. Others are chagrined that this year's commemoration ceremonies in Poland were strongly nationalistic and obscured the significance of the tragedy for the Jewish people.

The Smithsonian's Air and Space Museum had to cancel its interpretive exhibit of the Enola Gay, the plane that dropped the atomic bomb on Hiroshima, because it wasn't nationalistic enough for patriotic Americans. The plane will be shown, but alone and without comment. The exhibit had tried to give both sides of the issue, pointing out that the Americans started the nuclear era and the Japanese were victims, rather than depicting the Japanese threat and the magnitude of projected losses had the bomb not been dropped.

During the apparently inexorable events themselves, could a different course have been charted? Is it also too late for medicine to reclaim its rightful place in history? To remain powerful and independent, with patients who control their own destinies by choosing freely from physicians whose agendas include only their own best efforts at patient care?

Only if patients' own money ceases to be confiscated by insurance schemes and/or government and can be used fully in their own choices of doctors and venues. This would reflect a valid, real marketplace.

The so-called "medical market" of today's scene is a distortion, one in which an aspirin "costs" $5.00, and physicians are paid by the care they don't give ("capitation"). The term "capitated lives" is used in an attempt to impart seriousness to a business entity's activities. In reality, saving lives remains in the hands of skilled practicing physicians and nurses, not in a boardroom, where middlemen (or physicians-turned-middlemen) maximize their profits.

While the corporate, hospital and insurance domination of medicine has been called "market forces" and "capitalism finally at work in the medical field," it has been possible only because of legislation such as the 1972 HMO Act, the McCarran-Ferguson Act, and others, well-meaning, but causing severe market distortions. Patients and doctors could regain control with minimal legislative incentives, such as the Patient Protection Act and Health Saving Accounts, with public health, ongoing education, and with good will and cooperation by physicians and patients.

A doctor who joined the administration of a large organization smiled at me and said, "Yes, medicine and patients are suffering and will never be the same again, but think of the opportunity!" He and others will make the most of it, and will be on the other side of the rewriting of medical history. They will own the history, for they will have the power.

Most of us who understand the positive good in freedom and independence for doctor and patient will shake our heads and, like the shock and outrage we feel when the Holocaust is denied, we will be overcome with sadness for what was good and lasting, but is now going, and nearly gone.

CHAPTER FORTY-FOUR

Peace in the Streets: Safe at Last

Images are immeasurably important. This issue is about violence as public health problem. We prefer to call it "Peace in the Streets"—not as "Newspeak,"[1] but to help us visualize, image, and bring to pass the condition of peace in our communities.

Of course, it won't help to think we're safe until we are. But the constant mental picture and use of the word, *violence*, seems to give it an attention that *encourages* violence. Note how repeating the word evokes more violent feelings in yourself. *Peace, calm, tranquility*, the ability to move about as we please, the real personal autonomy to come and go, to accomplish what we wish, or to do nothing if that's our choice—in other words, to be *free*—is the image that must be gently, peaceably but pervasively reinfused into our common psyche.

Images are so important that many still believe the truism, popularized in the 1980s, "perception is reality." By this was meant that the only important thing was the bottom line impression—not how you *are* but how people think you are; not what is, but what seems to be.

How far from this is the 19th century poet Alice Cary's idea that, "True worth is in being, not seeming"—meaning that gradually doing some good, is better than just "seeming" to do it.

Many researchers have set out to prove scientifically that depicting violence begets violence. Folk wisdom goes both ways: that watching violent sports, combat, movies, etc., fulfills needs that may allow outlet for pent-up

---

1   In 1949, George Orwell wrote "Nineteen Eighty Four," a futuristic account of a "Big Brother," authoritarian government where everything was renamed its opposite, and history was rewritten to suit those in power.

feelings, thereby preventing individual acts of violence, or that copycat instincts encourage individuals to repeat what they see. There is research on the subject—it is not new, and it favors the idea that violent acts *do* follow after observing violence.

But those in control of media and government have little incentive to stress those studies. There is a "Catch 22" (from Joseph Heller's book by that name, a damned-if-you-do-and-if-you-don't premise makes solutions impossible.) The catch is: many people need and want the continuation of the violence for very practical reasons of self-interest. What would the military do without war? What would the cops do without killers to catch? What would trauma surgeons do without gunshot and knife wounds?

But this bland acceptance as normal should *not* be accepted by ordinary citizens. We are innocent bystanders and victims, even though each time we buy or choose violent "entertainment," we become unwitting, brainwashed complicitors.

There are many other people who benefit. Security companies depend on people's fears of crime to sell their wares. Makers of guns and bullets (some say regulate bullets strictly and it won't matter how many guns are out there), and bullet-proof vests have vested interests. Radio, TV and newspapers report briskly on every last act of criminal activity in the community in the guise of the public's right to know. They forget that we also have a right to know of the thousand acts of kindness, generosity and forgiveness occurring daily all around us, perhaps enhanced—as the media can do so well—by dramatic, first-hand, you-are-there presentations which excite our sensibilities As physician-citizens we must join the rest of the non-vested public in our mutual self-interest to live in peace and real security. Ways must be found not to blame those who enable the violence cascade, but to help them to see why purposeful diversion of their presently-lucrative activities into more productive directions will improve everyone's lives, just as the decline of smoking in this country—effected by a determined, enlightened populace led by medicine's luminaries—is convincing tobacco farmers to plant other crops, and tobacco companies to diversify.

My running partner and I started out at 6:00 AM as the moon set. We have felt perfectly safe doing this for over two years. As we finished the run she asked, "Did you see yesterday's paper? I can't believe how awful it is—the crime in this place." True, I had been mugged one night four years ago in front of my own house, but when I pointed out to her how safe we felt, how beautiful and peaceful the streets were, what a lovely run we just had, she decided it's not so bad after all.

Most of us sense that we're not as *unsafe* as the current statistics would imply, and that most people are peaceful, helpful and good. The hype and constant coverage of anomalous, bizarre behavior may be out of sync with real goals of change and nurture of solutions, and is unworthy of our attention—especially when it leads to more unwanted behavior.

This is a nation-wide, world-wide, age-old problem. Miami gets attention because of tourism. We have the chance to be a prototype of a call to action to reverse the violence, to create lasting peace via a creative, unified public health approach aimed at root causes, helped by our friends in law, in enforcement, in education, and in the media. We must recreate the excitement that images of peace and prosperity evoke so that, even as we face and fix the aberrant forces causing our pain and falsely exciting our imagination toward violence instead of peace, our best and most creative citizens will turn their faces away from the carnage and into the light.

It will take an inner change of attitude of the entire community. We physicians can help lead the way, with a can-do approach, since sooner or later, we touch the lives of everyone.

My image of Miami is one of sweet, spreading fingers of peace—the sultry sun and lapping sea, bright and growing greenery and mirrored moonlit nights. I grew up with these, and with peaceful people who were no less exciting because they did not exalt violence.

There were certain elements, even then, of criminality, and undercurrents of evil, as there can be anywhere. But the net effect was peace, and we were safe in the streets. These picture perfect postcard dreams can again be our reality.

CHAPTER FORTY-FIVE

The Biology and Genetics of Violence and Criminality

Physicians and others interested in physiology and behavior tend to wonder if violence has a biological basis. The topic would seem to need a prominent place in the study and understanding of such an important cause of death and disability. But considering the political events of this century, the inequities regarding under classes, and the feared discriminatory use such information may promote, many groups and persons are wary about uncovering knowledge in this area.

Specifically, a five-year, $400 million program planned by Louis W. Sullivan, MD, (an increase of $30 million/year) gave five-percent of its budget to fund "biological research," including studies of hormones and neurotransmitters linked to aggressive behavior in animal and humans. This part of the study was cancelled because Dr. Frederick K. Goodwin compared monkey violence and sexuality to jungle-like behavior within cities.[1]

A conference to be held at the University of Maryland, "Genetic Factors in Crime: Findings, Uses and Implications" was postponed for similar reasons. But the National Academy of Sciences called for more research in its report, "Understanding and Preventing Violence."

At the National Medical Association, a group of largely Black physicians, a plenary session was held on "Violence Reduction in the African-American Community: A prescription for Action." A Black political scientist, Ronald

---

[1] Horgan, J.; "Science and the Citizen: Genetics and Crime," *Scientific American.* February 1993. p. 24-29 2

Walters, PHD, objected strongly to the "medicalization" of what appeared to him to be a social and economic problem, and not a public health problem.[2]

But Black physicians on the panel, while admitting the reality of social factors, agreed that better surveillance, identification of risk factors, and targeted interventions were needed. These are precisely the methods of public health models.

Those embracing the scientific ethos tend to hold that the search for truth supplants all other considerations. Those who know too well the cruel uses to which adverse information can be put may judge that justice outweighs truth.

Truth might not "make you free." It could shackle individuals with a yoke of prejudgment. A more loving society might aver that a genetic, hormonal or biological flaw is a handicap for which we should have tolerance. The rigid obverse questions whether such flaws should be bred out of existence, or be forcibly, chemically altered, or not be allowed to live. Fears of such consequences can block fruitful and liberating research.

Just for simplistic example, since ninety-percent of violence is by young men in all societies is it not plausible that abnormal hormonal variation may be found to play a role in aberrant impulsive behavior, and might it not be harmlessly treated? Lack of faith bordering on anger causes disenchanted persons to suspect that research will not be well interpreted and used by society.

That same alienation can trigger rage leading to violence, whether or not biological variables are also involved. Thoughtful science with societal safeguards could sort out causes and effects.

---

2   Skolnick, A.A. ; "NMA seeks prescription to end violence," JAMA 270:183-4. Sept. 15, 199.

CHAPTER FORTY-SIX

Forensic Medicine and the Future

The Forensic Future

The application of medical science to legal problems is the definition of forensic medicine, also termed medical jurisprudence. The areas involved are usually paternity, insanity, injury, or death by violence. Even birth and death certificates are included.

The sordid job of picking up the pieces after crimes, accidents or other violent or suspicious means of meeting death is the picture most people have of the Medical Examiner's (coroner's) role. This is only a small part. With new research, the present role could expand to include work on prevention and treatment of criminal and asocial behavior.

The recent common wisdom is that there are no evil people, only evil deeds. You're not bad; you did a bad thing. This is fine for bringing up kids so that they can learn what the good things are while maintaining their self-esteem, even though they did one bad thing. But once that kid is past bringing up, and continues a pattern of misdeeds, what then? When does an evil person become recognized as truly evil, and what does he have to do (how many, how heinous, how senseless the crimes?) to gain the title? The belief, based in some but not all religions, that even the most evil can repent and thereby gain redemption clouds our willingness to apply the label "evil" to a person.

Recently, a killer, who had been sentenced to life imprisonment without parole in 1969, was granted a pardon in Pennsylvania in July, 1994. He proceeded to commit serial rapes and murders in 1994 in New York. After the fact, with ample agonizing blame for his release passed around to all involved, he was labelled a sociopath and a loner. It was admitted that the behavior could have been predicted had the system taken the time to examine him properly, even with current knowledge.

The idea exists, possibly based in fact, that people capable of such deeds are indeed afflicted with a pathological condition, almost by definition (the doing of the act defines their pathology, since the act itself is pathological), and therefore can no more be held responsible than diabetics or an epileptics.

One of the most famous epileptics of literary history, who served time in a Siberian penal colony, was Fyodor Dostoevsky, the great Russian novelist. He grappled with the subjects of good, evil, crime, punishment, and the pathology in human life. His own father was a military surgeon and a cruel despot, so heinous and hated that he was murdered by his own peasants. This had a profound effect upon the son. Dostoevsky's insights into the human character culminated in his masterpiece, *The Brothers Karamazov,* in which may be found a gamut of behaviors and motivations, spanning nearly all human activities and urges, good and evil.

Were Dostoevsky to have had today's technology in crime-solving and mental and physical disease diagnosis, his insights and conclusions might have been different. The ability to spot and treat conditions which afflicted some of the characters might have changed his stories. Who knows but what an enhanced use of measurements of hormones, epinephrine, neuro-transmitters and other yet-unknown brain and blood-levels in anti-social and asocial individuals may allow us to define and treat the criminal state, much as we have been able to treat the "insane" (schizophrenic, psychotic).

Yet the common, "normal" characteristics of the human condition (better understood by writers than by scientists), the seven deadly "sins," will always afflict the human character. Given lack of dominance of the seven less-exciting virtues, these rogue traits can break through to be motivation enough to commit crime.

Many persons get a sense of thrill from the chase, the risk, the dangers of near catch, the chance of capture. These are not peculiar to criminals; we all have such urges. Children's games and adult sports are variants of the concept. There appears to be a thin barrier between this type of arousal and that of a sexual type. There may be a gray area between "normal" and the spillover into pathological behavior. Aberrant and forbidden sexual behavior can produce even stronger, yet similar, effects. Both are highly sought compulsively, as fulfilling if not pleasurable sensations. How close these pleasure "centers" are to the areas which perceive sexual arousal and activity, even in normals, has not been answered. With the advent of PET scanners and other ways of measuring functional brain chemistry, there should be information forthcoming which perhaps can reveal causation of some of the more sordid crimes and their pathological triggers.

Figuring out who killed whom and with what weapon is one of the more dramatic and riveting activities with which forensic doctors are concerned. Murder itself is fascinating to non-murderers chiefly because of a grudging respect for the perpetrator: he/she has done something which the non-criminal is unable to do. Like walking a tightrope, dangling from a ledge, or playing a flawless sonata, most of us have no skill for what it takes. We are incapable of and could not kill someone in cold blood, or even in self-defense. We are possessed of a conscience and an empathy which stops us in our tracks.

A powerful counterbalance, such as protection of our young or of ourselves, would need to be operating for the deed to be done. So the perpetrator—not just of murder but of lesser, even civil crimes seems to deserve attention and awe. The criminal has power to act in a way denied the "normal" person. How else to explain the fascination "good" people have with evil deeds and their doers? There may also be an element of "thrill," available to the criminal, denied to the non-criminal, but reached vicariously by the fascinated spectator.

Thus it is the pathology—the deviation from the norm—that grabs the attention of everyone. It is the urge to know why—the mechanism of disease—that fascinates. These are merely the same moving forces behind the physician's early and ongoing interest in medicine: wondering why and looking for reasons, then attempting to fix the problem.

Meticulously-obtained medical facts and their application to cases lead to identification and elucidation of crucial elements in criminal and civil litigation. Theoretically, this knowledge should lead to justice for all. There is an implied mission, best exemplified by the etched letters over the doorway of the Supreme Court of the United States in Washington, DC: "We who labor here seek only truth."

Unfortunately, the wished-for scenario does not always ensue. Despite the most carefully prepared cases, with facts at hand, justice does not always happen. Perhaps medical examiners seek only truth, but lawyers may not, notwithstanding their etched-in-stone mottos. Lawyers seek to represent their clients and win. The theory is that the truth will emerge, given the vigor of the adversary system, which is said to allow both sides to thrive. The faith implicit is that the best (most truthful) will prevail, because a jury of peers will render judgment based on fact alone, as instructed. But the best in court does not always reveal the truth. Even many lawyers will agree that the method lacks fairness, and point out that it's the worst system—except for all the others.

Forensic science may help sort out ethically-befuddled stances. It may come to seem less unethical to treat with hormones or other chemicals an aggressive, hostile pedophile (yes, involuntarily if necessary), than to release him to victimize yet another child. Medical jurisprudence could be researching and recommending intervention in similar cases. If, by enhanced forensic medical techniques, our certainty of not incarcerating innocent persons improves, we will be less hesitant to believe that many common crimes are in the category of "extraordinary circumstance," warranting imposing unwanted treatments on prisoners whose civil liberties are often now respected more than those of their past or future victims. Medical doctors need to liberalize, with more thought to victims than to criminals, their definitions of "appropriate candidates" for treatment. Prisons should be clinical and social laboratories, and prisoners fair subjects for humane study.

The use of medical jurisprudence to help attorneys and judges settle cases for accused persons is a worthy one. If truth is reached more often than not, it also serves the public. Data accumulated from cases, along with newer approaches to mechanisms and valid theories of causation, may allow for new understanding. With more certainty and better organization, sound decisions could be made when rehabilitation is likely to succeed.

When, for some, the pathology (the person) is incurable with our present store of treatment options, permanent solutions without wasteful, disastrous attempts at failed remedies, should ensue. Laws could suggest certain treatments for certain crimes, so that criminals would know in advance what treatments would be sure and swift based on medical evidence and inference from the nature of the crime.

This expanded role of forensic medicine would seem to be a logical direction for the skills of forensic medical doctors and researchers, guiding the legal arm into the scientific approach to solving the quadruple problems of prevention, diagnosis, treatment and rehabilitation. If others among sociologists, criminologists, practicing personal physicians, university professors or even prison physicians are also in a position to fill this role, they should. But no one has the unique combination of skills required. This enhanced interpretation of the definition of forensic medicine fits a future which commands creative applications of medical science to legal problems.

CHAPTER FORTY-SEVEN

Late Blooming Roses

When we moved to Coral Gables twenty-five years ago, we were greeted by an elderly widower bearing beautiful roses from his prize-winning rose-garden. He sold his house a few years ago at the age of ninety-five to marry his girlfriend; caring for his house and garden was just then becoming hard for him.

I was eight when I learned to do a back-bend, holding onto the cross-bar of our backyard swing. My grandmother was visiting the day I let go and could do it alone. She came out to watch my new trick. I remember imprinting my thoughts so I would remember later, seeing her slow-moving, ponderous frame watching my lithe mobility with a certain longing. I was pondering with new insight the difference between her and me, not just the age. I said to myself, I will never get so overweight and stiff that I can't do this. If I keep it up until I become a grandmother myself, why shouldn't I still be able to do it?

Once, when we got a brand-new car, my son, aged four, sat unusually quietly, staring at the door and the seats, stroking them with his hands, thinking deep thoughts. After a while, he looked up quizzically and asked, "How do things get old?" I was hard-put to describe to a four-year-old, the gradual ravages of time, wear and tear, on people or cars. I am not as stiff as my grandmother at her age, but I can no longer do the same back-bend.

My grandmother could do much more than a back-bend; she could endear my childish heart to her. She must have been an important source for me of a lifelong attraction and patience for old people, their wisdom, stories and points of view.

We often hear that our children are our future. But for each of us, it seems more clear that our parents are our future. Living or dead, they reflect our own selves in but a few years. If they are alive, they have the one clear advantage of age: knowing that they made it that far. We might not be so lucky. Where is it written which decade of one's life is most vital, most valuable to an individual? Some live into their eighties or nineties, only to find their most fulfilling experience of all, either interpersonal or occupational. The love of one's life is not restricted by age. Many have married for the first time or the first good time. Others have pursued new careers or broken new ground. Some are content to revel in memories or to live each day. There are late bloomers everywhere. Stereotypes and rules don't apply now, and maybe never did. There are unusual arrangements and contingencies, especially now that many live longer and better, thanks partly to us in the helping professions.

A paradox of medical care for the aged is that just when they need it most, society is conspiring to deny it to them. Many elderly have their priorities straight and realize that medical attention is worth as much or much more than many material objects, for which most people pay willingly, having budgeted and saved. Yet the Medicare system sets out to deny individual elderly the right to contract with a physician to render more superior care than that of a minimalist system in which government foots the bill and manages the money. Any person should have the right to purchase what they please; but—as in Canada, where you can buy a CAT scan for your dog but not for yourself—Medicare rules specifically try to prohibit that basic right, in a misguided egalitarianism. As physicians, we need to be skilled at imagining—for our patients—what it's like to be ill or disabled by age, for aging will inevitably mean some disability, even if it's just hearing loss, general slowdown, or wrinkles.

I have been doing a series of videotapes of some of the elderly in my practice for use in educating the young doctors rotating through as preceptees in family practice. They often have no idea of the fascinating, ongoing vigor of these wonderful people, nor what they have learned or endured, and what they can teach. They get to see them "gorked out," at their worst, sick, helpless, and sometimes crotchety. Such patients' lack of personal appeal is legend in cruel medical novels and first-person accounts of so-called humorists, who tell (and sell) all about hospital life. Some of us never laughed—at least not at the patients' expense, but perhaps to relieve our own anxiety and desperation, knowing that soon, we will be in their places.

Writing in *Newsweek's* "My Turn" column, a young deaf woman poignantly expressed the idea that, "we're all just temporarily abled, and every one of us, if we live long enough, will become disabled in some way. Those of us who have gotten there first can tell you how to cope with…ways of holding a book, opening a door and leaning on a crutch all at the same time. And what it's like to give up in despair on Thursday, then begin all over again on Friday, because there's no other choice—and because roses are beginning to bud in the garden."[1]

---

[1]   Nicolette Toussaint, *Newsweek*; May 23, 1994; page 10.

CHAPTER FORTY-EIGHT

"Doctor, Doctor—Will I Die?" ("Yes, My Dear, and so Will I.")

In the work of medicine, the poetry all around sometimes escapes us, for lack of time or tuning-in. Especially in these days of unwelcome distraction from our only purpose (taking care of sick people—and its corollary keeping them well), we may tend not to nourish the very qualities on which depend our ability to practice the art of medicine.

Two poets took different tacks: one begged his father not to go gently into that good night, and exhorted him to "rage against the dying of the light."[1] The other was still a teenager when he wrote that when one is ready to approach the grave, one could "wraps the drapery of his couch…about him, and lie down to pleasant dreams." [2]

Yet both Dylan Thomas and William Cullen Bryant were equally optimists in their opposite views. Then there was the poet with the humorous outlook that he's just bound—as in the song—away.[3] And he may return if dissatisfied with what he learned, having died. Robert Frost also said he would like to go as a "swinger of birches, which he did in his boyhood, bending toward heaven and being set down again.[4]

My father made light of his dire disease—whenever someone asked how he was doing he would say, "I'm sick in bed with two nurses." (In those days, that was neither harassment nor sexism, just cute.) When he died of heart disease just before my son was born, I was disconsolate and wrote a eulogy for us both.[5] Many years later my mother penned her own succinct summary in one line.[6]

There may be some truth to the notion that doctors (and other medical people) may be non-randomly self-selected with perhaps even more problems dealing with death than others. The study of medicine, itself, can be an attempt to ward off coming closer to death and disease, as though by knowing all about it, one could control or avoid it. One can put off the profound, ultimate questions of "why?" by asking and knowing with enviable near certainty the answers to "how?" Saying he died of pulmonary edema, and knowing all the mechanisms, defers the more unanswerable questions—"why him, why now?" and "why life and death?"

Apart from our personal, intimate losses, our brushes with the deaths of our patients involve another type of investment of self. It may feel emotionally draining, the closer we allow ourselves to get. But it needn't take anything away from us, unless we fail to understand the secret strength it lends.

Whatever we give of ourselves is held closely. It is not dissipated but is returned in overfull measure. Even when acts are unknown, unrecognized and unappreciated, as thousands of behind-the-scenes efforts often are, they come back to us in genuine, reality-based satisfaction and peace.

So pick your poet: we can go kicking and screaming, or full of peace, or jauntily singing songs and playing games; fearful or faithful, depressed or enlightened, seeing an end or a beginning, trying to hang in tenaciously or moving aside gracefully—however one fancies one will go, go one must. And who is there when it happens? For our patients, very often, it is we physicians who ease the way. We can hope that our flexible skills and compassion will allow us to meet patients on their own special turf, meshing well with their own long held beliefs and intentions.

But we wonder sometimes, who will be there for us as we were for them? Who will ease our path? The answer: each time we help someone else, we help ourselves, so that when our time comes it will be easy, so easy. Whether someone is there or not won't matter much, though it would be nice to have the same solace we gave so often. Whether in true belief, or in willing suspension of disbelief, we can accept that all who were helped by us also helped us, their spirits stay with us, and remain to ease our way. They have not forgotten. Nor will we.

Endnotes

1   "Do Not Go Gently Into That Good Night" by Dylan Thomas; From "The Poems of Dylan Thomas," published by New Directions. Copyright © 1952, 1953 Dylan Thomas. Copyright © 1938, 1939, 1943, 1946, 1971 New Directions Publishing Corp., NY, NY.

2   "Thanatopsis," by William Cullen Bryant... "By an unfaltering trust, approach thy grave/ Like one who wraps the drapery of his couch/ About him, and lies down to pleasant dreams."

3   "Away!" by Robert Frost... "I'm—bound—Away!/ And I may return/ If dissatisfied/ With what I learn/ From having died."

4   "Birches," by Robert Frost... "I'd like to get away from earth awhile/ And then come back to it and begin over."

5   "Eulogy For Daddy And Me"—Buried nowhere/ You are everywhere./ Having no grave,/ I cannot visit/ Except in memory/ Or in every leaf.// The life you gave me/ I am giving back / Slowly—As my son matures/ (You've not seen him but he has your name)/ As you gave yours./ You are not the only one who ever died/ Nor I who ever cried./ I would feel sad/ But that you had/ No more control/ Over cycles than I./ So—instead of only sad/ I feel myself already/ Dead./ And mourn for me/ Ahead.

6   "Life is a dress-rehearsal for which there will never be an opening night." by Esther Granat.

CHAPTER FORTY-NINE

Swan Song

Once, long ago, it was believed that swans were mute, withholding all wisdom, destined to sing one song only, at death.[1]

From that image came the general meaning: the last words and efforts of those whose work is done.[2] It has come to imply not a prior withholding of voice, but a leave-taking, a farewell.

Being an essayist for *Miami Medicine* has allowed me to comment on many concerns and projects. This issue devoted to "Music and Medicine," is my last as editor, my swan song. We are privileged to have as co-editor for this issue, Dr. Robert Gower, an exceptionally fine pianist, accompanist and composer. He accompanies the University Civic Chorale in which I have sung for the past twenty-five years. The melding of musical and medical concerns is evident in the fascinating articles in this issue.

Music is my medicine. I sang before I walked or talked. When I was a child on Miami Beach during the war, the army took over all the hotels, and drilled in the residential streets right in front of my house. My first images are of singing all their songs, running alongside. In high school I played in the band, sang in the chorus and participated in operettas and musical plays. A band scholarship paid my tuition at the University of Miami.

My sisters and my children also took part musically, in school and in other organizations. None of us were stars, but I credit music with developing self-confidence, discipline, responsibility and sensitivity in all of us. I credit music with putting us in touch with a universal language.

Participating as one small element of a chorus or band submerges the self, but also joins the self into a larger truth. It matters, as one vote matters, and it is a heavy responsibility. Each performed work has a life and time of its own, a rise and a fall. It is learned, rehearsed, performed, and becomes a reverberating memory. Sometimes the past feelings associated with its unique life are resurrected many years later, when the same work is performed again, though the new production always takes on its own personality.

Music is a survival skill. It is a cry of faith, though all seems lost (*Alleluia, Shma Yisroel*). It calls to arms, it buries the dead, it carries a bride down the aisle. It lulls babies to sleep, and parents to dream. It prays and curses; it is reverent and salacious; it dances and dirges; it frolics and sighs. It makes work go effortlessly. It affects the autonomic nervous system, depending both on its physical stimuli (vibration, tone, pitch, rhythm) and its intellectual content (religious, patriotic, story-telling, emotional, romantic, traditional, spiritual, modern, exhortatory, commercial, functional). It is one of the essentials to take with you on a desert island.

In music, as in medicine, there is the striving for perfection. Sometimes, we come close. Sometimes we save or improve lives. Always, we try. The lost chord is a concept of fleeting perfection when all comes together in complete harmony. A lone organist who found it once, searches worldwide to hear it again, and imagines that only with death may it be found again, in the most common concept of perfectibility: heaven. A chorus of angels dominates any heavenly metaphor. Music was nurtured in all religions. Music is part of humankind's spiritual life, even those who consider themselves most secular—especially they, for music may be one of their only touches with spiritual feelings.

Insofar as physicians must grapple constantly with delaying or meeting death, the blissful chorus, not the grim reaper might be cultivated as our preferred image. In Robert Frost's poem, "Come In," the poet came to the edge of the woods at dusk, and heard thrush music. It was too dark inside the woods for the thrush to fly to another perch, though it still could sing. The sun that had died, still lived in the song, which was a call to come into the woods and lament, a metaphor for entering the darkness of death. When our choral director, who chose the Duruflé Requiem which we recently performed, said that he wanted this work played at his funeral, I surmised he also meant he would like to die with this gorgeous music singing in his last breath, ringing in his mind's ear. Psychologists are learning now that it is possible to program and direct our own dreams. We arrange the joyous music that marks milestones in our lives. Perhaps we can learn to plan our last images. If we could, there would always be music, our own swan song.

Endnotes

1   The Silver Swan (Orlando Gibbons 1583—1625) The silver swan who, living, had no note, When death approach'd, unlock'd her silent throat: Leaning her breast against the reedy shore, Thus sang her first and last, and sang no more. Farewell all joys, O death come close mine eyes; More geese than swans now live, more fools than wise. The A Capella Singer, Edited by H. Clough-Leighter; E.C. Schirmer Music Co. Boston Mass., 1936.

2   swan song n.[trans. of G. *schwanenlied*] 1: a song of great sweetness formerly thought to be uttered by the swan just before its death 2 : a farewell appearance or final act or pronouncement (the swan song of a chivalry which died in the century before—*New Republic*) (before turning over the gavel delivered the swan song as chairman of the board); specif: the last work (as of an author or composer) Webster's *Third New International Dictionary*, Unabridged, Encyclopedia Britannica, 1976.

Epilogue: Fulfilling the Circle

The young woman in the red Chevette died. I rode with her in the ambulance to the ER, attempting to bag her. She never really made it, even to the emergency room. Everyone knew she was dead at the scene, especially me, but all had hoped.

Though the futile, heroic attempts were in vain, they served their human and humane function of fooling us into thinking we did something—at least that we cared enough to try. The bystanders all felt that, although they were only onlookers.

For me, although I had been through many emergencies in my medical training up to that point, as well as several while on travels, none had been so close, so devastating and so heart-wrenching, not to mention so physically intimate.

I must have endured a variant of post-traumatic stress disorder for a while after, and even now, in reliving and rewriting it, I begin to weep with sadness for the life snatched away, and for all the lives we're trying to save and can't. We all know our attempts are just as futile—everyone dies. But few are so immediate and so sudden as that day against the tree.

These kinds of episodes are delicately balanced by the real, less bombastic, yet often successful dramas that play out in our offices daily, as we quietly and enthusiastically influence our patients and, as workmanlike, we do our jobs. While despair and feelings of uselessness are one response, a counter-response is just as strong, and more fun. It is an effect of heightened resolve, of new faith in the mission of medicine—which is more than just a job—and in the symmetrical, balanced beauty and poetry of medicine. It is an effect of heightened ambition toward the ideal of becoming real doctors.

9 798535 063058